Now What?

A Guide to the Gifts and Challenges of Aging

To learn more about this book and the authors, please visit:
www.HealthyAgingBook.com

Cover design and illustration by Rick Nease
www.RickNeaseArt.com

Published by
Front Edge Publishing
42807 Ford Road, Suite 234
Canton, MI

Front Edge Publishing books are available for discount bulk purchases for
events, corporate use and small groups. Special editions, including books with
corporate logos, personalized covers and customized interiors are available
for purchase. For more information, contact Front Edge Publishing at info@
FrontEdgePublishing.com

This book is dedicated to the elders of Detroit,
whose stories have inspired us,
and have revealed how much work remains to be done.

Contents

Praise for *Now What?*

Now What? is a rarity as a book in that it delivers exactly what it promises: comprehensive guidance to the gifts and challenges of aging. This book recognizes that aging offers many forks in the road for both individuals and communities. One fork in the road can easily lead to such unnecessary experiences as loneliness, insecurity, a lack of self-care, unpreparedness, as well as a failure to adequately view both one's history and present value as a person. The other fork in the road honors relationship-building, financial preparedness, improving home security, and the opportunity to entertain new skills, finally having the space to embrace different types of activities, and a chance to embrace one's new place in life. When this happens, as was said of Ezra Pound later in his life: "He listened more eloquently, instead of talking eloquently."

Another amazing feature of this brief volume is its ability to address both caregivers and those in need of support, fellowship and aid to improve quality of life. If you only skim the lists of practical information provided in each chapter, you will be so much better prepared to live a full life more sagely and enjoyably with less unnecessary worry, and guide others in the process as well. As I turned the final pages in this book, I thought to myself: How could the contributors know so much and be able to share it in a way that was so enriching to both individuals and communities if they avail themselves of the information and suggested steps offered? In addition to these questions, I also felt a profound sense of gratitude for the contributors' successful efforts. *Now What?* is truly a gift I hope you will embrace and encourage others to do so as well. What a positive change such a careful reading of the material can make.

Dr. Robert J. Wicks, the author of *Perspective: The Calm within the Storm and Bounce: Living the Resilient Life*, advises groups on resilient living around the world.

Now What? is a comprehensive how-to manual for successful aging and living a full life. This book is packed with helpful advice, tips, links and recommendations for those in their later years, their families and their caretakers. Written in an accessible and easy-to-read style, you can jump right to a topic or chapter of interest or read the book from start to finish. However you read it, keep this book handy for use now and in the future. It's a book that we all need.

Wayne E. Baker is the Robert P. Thome Professor of Business Administration & Faculty Director at the Center for Positive Organizations, University of Michigan Ross School of Business.

This is a very wise book—one that I wish I had back when I was "pastor of visitation" at a Presbyterian church and visited 30 seniors each month. I would recommend that churches and community groups give two books to each family—one for the senior and one for a friend or relative—so that an entire family can read this book together.

That's in keeping with one of the valuable pieces of wisdom in this book: "Organize a team to help in the care of a senior." Far too often, the care of a senior falls to one or two people, but if a team is established, this is extended to welcome more people into a healthy and sustainable community.

Lucille Sider is a clinical psychologist and clergywoman in Chicago who is the author of *Light Shines in the Darkness: My Healing Journey Through Sexual Abuse and Depression*.

For generations Benjamin Spock's classic *Baby and Child Care* provided calm, reassuring guidance for those entering the uncharted territory of parenthood. In a similarly wise, clear fashion, *Now What? A Guide to the Gifts and Challenges of Aging* gently illuminates our paths as once again new chapters unfold before us.

Rabbi Bob Alper is the author of *Thanks. I Needed That.* and *Life Doesn't Get Any Better Than This*.

How often have you asked yourself: Now what? I wonder about that every day. As I travel along my life journey, I continue to check in with myself and think about what I need, what is important to me, how I contribute to my community and where I want to go next. I have really embraced aging and each decade brings new revelations and opportunities to create a life that suits me now. Keeping things simple, connecting with folks who accept me, investing in my overall health and wellbeing, and pursuing my passions have allowed me to thrive in many areas of my life.

This book offers wonderful resources and tools to answer questions and point you in the right direction as you consider your next steps and move into a new season of life. The guide offers thoughtful and poignant information to help you create your own plan for supporting your personal journey. Each and every one of us has unique gifts, strengths and talents that benefit others. Each cycle of our lives produces questions and situations that call for new information. Each of us has questions on what is best for ourselves and those we love. You will find help as you try to answer those questions in these pages. And remember: Your life experience and wisdom you have collected is a beautiful gift to share!

Shaun Taft is a Macro Social Worker who helps nonprofits improve service to individuals and their communities.

Now What? could be subtitled, "Finding Meaning in Later Life." Many Americans struggle when earlier roles—such as parenting and work—are gone. This is a helpful, comprehensive guide to aging. It offers positive options in a culture that tends to view later life negatively. It is full of practical tips for everything from helping people discover what is really important to them, to downsizing, caregiving and care receiving, nurturing relationships, hospice, funeral planning—and everything in between. This is a valuable resource for those aging and for those who care about aging friends and family.

Carol Myers is a nationally known educator who leads workshops for families and congregations especially focusing on caring for the neediest in our communities.

As a pastor, this is the Bible I would want to give to retirees and the aging. In my churches I frequently gave Bibles to third graders and graduates, hoping it would speak to them as they matured. *Now What?* is an exceedingly wise guide for everyone maturing into the last third of their lives.

Over a dozen authors bring their compassion and expertise to the full range of experiences involved in aging. You get Dmitri Barvinok's practical help for creating a safe home and becoming internet savvy; Najah Bazzy's transcultural perspectives on nurturing and sharing our hard-won wisdom; Benjamin Pratt's always-tender encouragement to caregivers; and the Rev. Charles Ensminger's reassuring guidance for the anxious task of funeral planning. Their stories, questions, quotes and suggestions spark hope and optimism as you read through these brief-but-rich chapters.

I don't know where else you would find in one volume this sort of everyday help and spiritual sensitivity blended with such positive encouragement. That's why I say this truly is a "Good Book." As it points out multiple social, spiritual, physical, occupational, educational and creative pathways into the future, it truly has the potential to change your life—and the lives of those you love.

The Rev. Dr. Larry Buxton is the author of *Thirty Days With King David: On Leadership*.

I love this book. So many books for caregivers are too heavy to quickly scan and understand, and this one is different: precise and easy to apply. *Now What?* presents critical information with great clarity for those who are aging and experiencing multiple new facets of life in later years. This new book provides real and applicable strategies for expanding one's capacity to grow and create quality of life in the most difficult of times. The common-sense concepts are easy to understand and offer new ways to view personal and family dynamics. These experts remind readers to direct planning energies toward efforts that "improve health, well-being and the enjoyment of life" while providing key techniques that make these goals attainable.

Daphne Johnston is the founder of the Respite for All Foundation.

I am very impressed with this book, thanks to all the wonderful authors who contributed chapters. What I like best is that the material in this book is very helpful not only to seniors but also to those who live with and care for them. I am 74 years old now and I found many good ideas in the pages of this book that I'm going to use myself! This book confirms that Don Quixote was right. Be inspired to follow The Impossible Dream and don't see life like it is—but like it could be. So many people see "aging" as The End, where this transforming book reminds us that aging can be just The Beginning.

Now What? is full of helpful, pragmatic suggestions to improve the lives of seniors and to remind them that "You are not alone." This book reminds us all that aging well requires a systemic approach to our senior years. If we are intentional and deliberate about discovering the Gifts and Challenges of Aging, we can enjoy and succeed in life for years and years to come.

The Rev. Rodger Murchison is the author of *Guide for Grief: Help in surviving the stages of grief and bereavement after a loss*.

I began reading, *Now What?* from a singular point of view: my interest in what the this book describes as "Saging." Knowing the perils my own children and grandchildren face in their futures, I long to better understand my role in guiding them. I certainly found wise guidance for my role as a hope-filled and loving elder. However, I also found what I was not seeking; that being wisdom for understanding my limits as a sager, including the uncomfortable fact that my children and grandchildren exhaust me! At the moment, as a 71 year-old senior, I have more to give than I need to receive from the youngsters. But this season is too rapidly passing me by. *Now What?* has opened my eyes to what is required of me as one who both blesses and is blessed. Let it happen. Pay attention to what is happening. Do not resist what is happening. Let this book inform and support you on your way; share it with the ones who best care for you. I will.

The Rev. Ken Whitt is a pastor, spiritual director and the author of *God Is Just Love: Building Spiritual Resilience and Sustainable Communities for the Sake of Our Children and Creation*.

Foreword

I grew up in a multi-generational home. Even before I was born, my maternal grandparents lived with my family. Their lives were integrated into every fiber of my young life. When I was 7 and my parents built a new house, they thoughtfully designed a separate but connected living space to provide my grandparents privacy and a sense of independence for their late years.

As time passed and my grandparents aged, I had a front-row seat to watching my parents encourage and tenderly care for them. Looking back as an adult, I realize there must have been times of stress, but as a youth I only remember seeing grace, gratitude and perseverance in action. It was a remarkable opportunity for me to learn from two generations of family members who chose to walk alongside each other on the journey of aging. I am certain those early experiences helped shape who I am and why I am so passionate about encouraging older adults today as a writer and speaker on issues of aging faithfully.

My first book, *Living with Purpose in a Worn-Out Body*, was birthed in my own experiences as a caregiver for my parents in their elder years. Gratefully, they had learned well from my grandparents. They showed wisdom in planning for their own late life. They were unafraid to talk about end-of-life issues. They made sure that necessary financial and legal documents were updated and appropriately filed, making my role, and the role of my siblings, so much easier.

My older brother and sister were equally as devoted to our parents, but as the only adult child living within a short driving distance from our parents, I naturally assumed the primary responsibility for their daily care as their needs changed over time. It was during this season of transition that I first began to think about aging as a family affair. I had learned that any change in my aging parents' lives—a health emergency, not being able to drive, diminished mobility—had a reciprocal effect on my life. It was not a complaint. It was just reality.

Ten books and 12 years later, I have expanded my thinking about aging. Though it certainly is a family affair, I have come to realize that aging is also a community affair. With a fast-growing population of older adults, communities are struggling with how to help families with aging loved ones navigate the rocky landscape that comes with growing older.

I was reminded of that struggle a few years ago when I passed by a middle-aged man leaning up against the wall in an empty hallway of a hospital. It was obvious that he was highly stressed because he was muttering loudly to himself. I soon discovered that his mother had suffered a stroke and had to leave the hospital in three days. He was functioning in sheer panic, not knowing what to do first or where to turn as he tried to deal with all the ripple effects of his mother's health crisis. His thoughts turned to his aging father who had physical limitations of his own. What would happen to him? Soon it became evident that he was feeling pangs of regret for not having been more involved in his parents' care as they had aged.

I can only imagine how this middle-aged man's frame of mind might have been different if he would have had *Now What? A Guide to the Gifts and Challenges of Aging* long before his mother's medical crisis. Certainly, he would have been more prepared with this plethora of information at his fingertips.

It is true that every person's journey of aging is unique. That's why this book offers such a vast array of information on the most vital topics of aging. Drawing on the expertise and experiences of professionals involved in eldercare, this book will truly guide families through the uneven landscape of late life—and will point readers toward helpful answers for the question we all share, at some point in life: Now what?

Missy Buchanan

www.missybuchanan.com

Introduction

Each life is unique. But, as we age, we reach an almost universal moment of feeling overwhelmed. There is so much to figure out, so much to do, so much to decide. The problems and challenges snowball. One question leads to more. One "simple" slip and fall can transform an active, independent person into someone who needs fulltime assistance and care. Suddenly, we need to understand Medicare, Medicaid, spend-downs, home care, long-term care planning, advance directives, patient advocates …

The lists can go on and on.

As we age and as those we love age, we find ourselves asking, "Now what?" Mom has an Alzheimer's diagnosis—now what? Dad's vision is going—now what? My life partner is no longer able to manage our household finances—now what? I am almost 65 and want to retire—now what?

All of these are potentially overwhelming, life-changing questions. But, they also are opportunities—milestones when we must stop and ask ourselves, and those around us, to listen and be heard, to learn and to communicate clearly, to discover both the truth of the problems we may be facing—as well as the new doorways still opening ahead of us. Hence, the title of this book: *Now What? A Guide to the Gifts and Challenges of Aging.* Like so much of our human experience, as we approach life's autumn, there is darkness and light, sadness and joy, confusion and clarity. It is our hope that through the information included in these pages that aging will also be seen not just as a time of problems to be solved—but also as a time filled with gifts.

Whether you are contemplating your own aging or helping a loved one, we hope that this book will offer you guideposts on your journey. The authors within these pages share their collective wisdom and experiences in working with people just like you—people like all of us.

This book is for everyone. It is for the caregiver and for the care receiver. It is for the seasoned and for the novice. It is for those who are fear-laden and for those who are living their best lives. It is for those who need a starting point for the conversation and for those who need just a bit of guidance in their final decision-making. It is a book that is intended for everyone.

When this book invites "you" to look at ways "we" can respond to the aging process—our authors are intentionally welcoming everyone to accept these invitations. The "you" and "we" really represents all of "us"—care receivers and caregivers, family members, friends and professionals.

This book was written as a general introduction to the many topics covered in these chapters—practical, honest encouragement, based on the "best practices" professionals recommend today. These chapters are helpful orientations to these topics offered in a general way for all readers, not an exhaustive coverage of each issue. If you care to learn more, our authors provide many suggestions of where you might turn next.

It is our hope that this book will wind up worn, tattered and dog-eared, filled with notes and highlights as you pull it off the shelf, carry it around, discuss it with friends and use it on a regular basis.

We hope that you read it cover to cover, but also that you use it as a reference, finding particular passages that relate to what you are going through right now.

Finally, we invite you to help us continue to develop this book and helpful resources around it. Please visit www.HealthyAgingBook.

com to find more helpful materials. From the website, you can let us know what you found most helpful, what we missed, what we should update and expand—and how we can make future editions of the book even more helpful to all of the people who need this book, for themselves and for a loved ones.

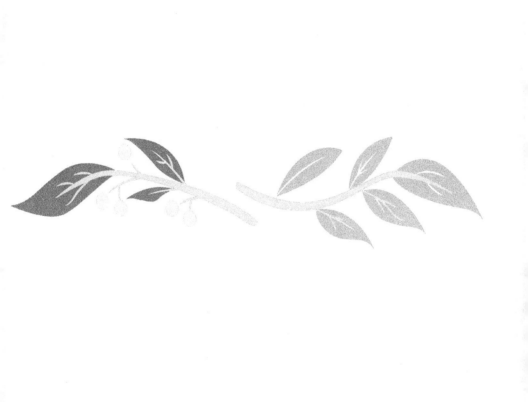

You Are Not Alone

Connecting in healthy ways with our community

In four words, the message of this book is: You are not alone.

Those four words echo throughout this book because isolation and exclusion are the two greatest threats to our health and well-being. In the pages of this book, you will learn dozens of ways people around us can help—if we reach out and welcome that assistance.

The fact that these issues are so threatening is no surprise after the many months of isolation during the COVID-19 pandemic. As we all recall, at the start of this global crisis, we hoped we would only need to stay in our homes for a few weeks. At first, many of us felt a bit of relief and perhaps excitement that the busyness of our lives would be replaced by some quiet time at home. Social engagements would not be honored, many of us would be working from home, our calendars were freeing up. We would all be hunkering down for a while, often with loved ones at home.

Then days rolled into weeks—and weeks into months. We longed for the ability to come and go as we pleased—to get our hair cut, to return to our houses of worship, to hug our friends and family. We moved from being alone to being lonely; from being socially isolated to feeling socially excluded. Our mental health was impacted not only by the anxiety and fear that come from living through a pandemic, but also by our lack of human connection.

A moment's reflection will allow us to translate our personal experiences during that time of self-isolation to the experiences of our aging friends, family members and neighbors.

For those who are beginning to experience some aging-related limitations, the slip into times of isolation and periods of loneliness may not have occurred as abruptly as the restrictions resulting from the pandemic. But the aging process often leads to a seemingly endless struggle with isolation and exclusion—a process that can deepen into a dangerous lack of emotional, physical and spiritual resources that can last not only for months, but for many years.

In her 1968 memoir, *The Measure of My Days*, analytical psychologist Florida Scott-Maxwell reveals her own mixed feelings in her journaling. One day, she wrote in frustration: "I wish a notebook could laugh." At times, she revels in the fact that she can waltz on her kitchen floor, noting that "This pleasure is for the old who live alone." At other times, she longs for connection. She describes the joy that comes through shared laughter, but also how exhausting it can be simply to spend time with other people. When she is with other people, she feels the need to ignore her physical pain, to do the mental work of creating connection with those in her presence, to wait on her guests. She finds this all quite tiring and wonders: Which is better—isolation or company?

The answer is that *both* isolation and company are needed. We need to feel human connection, but we also need quiet time. We need rest. We need time to process, to reflect, to focus on ourselves. As we age, it can take extra effort to hear everything that is happening around us. It takes physical and mental energy to overcome any pain and discomfort we are experiencing. After time with others, we need time to rest and rejuvenate, at any age.

The National Poll on Healthy Aging (www.healthyagingpoll.org), conducted by the University of Michigan and involving more than 2,000 50- to 80-year-olds, publishes monthly reports on a variety of aging issues. Its March 2019 Loneliness and Health report found that one-third of study respondents felt a lack of companionship and 27% felt isolated from others, with women, those who weren't working, those with lower incomes, and those who lived alone more likely to report such feelings. It is interesting to note that respondents with children living with them were also more likely to report feeling a lack of companionship or isolation from others. Living with someone else does not insulate us from loneliness.

It is important that all of us have someone with whom to connect on a regular basis. For those who live with other people, that check-in likely occurs naturally. For those who live alone, we may need to set up a structure for "wellness checks." These calls can be conducted by someone who you know or set up with an agency like the local Area Agency on Aging (eldercare.acl.gov/Public/Index.aspx) or other eldercare service provider. These calls can be quite brief, just ensuring that the person on the receiving end picks up the phone, or they can be long chats about the events of the day and days gone by. In any case, they are an important touchpoint to make sure that those living alone aren't in crisis or to help them get assistance if needed.

Here are some tips for overcoming feelings of isolation. You will discover that many of these ideas are explored in more depth as you read more chapters of this book. But this is a great quick inventory of the many options we have in coping with isolation. You may even want to share this with a friend who is lonely as a way to spark a healthy conversation.

- Recognize that human connection is important for physical and mental health
- Volunteer
- Participate in community groups
- Engage in a faith community
- Schedule regular time with loved ones
- Walk through the community and interact with neighbors
- Share a meal
- Find the right balance of time with others and time alone
- Phone a friend
- Try social media
- Eat healthy food, be physically active, and get enough sleep

Keep in mind that the right amount and kinds of interactions are going to be different for each individual and will likely vary from day to day.

If feelings of loneliness turn into a looming dark cloud that hangs in your world day after day, it's time to have a talk with a doctor. There are many effective treatments for depression. If there is an urgent need for mental health services, the national Substance Abuse and Mental Health Services Administration's National Helpline is 1-800-662-HELP (4357).

Our Allies

Organizing a successful team

Millions of Americans tackle the challenges of aging on their own. If they suddenly need a caregiver at some crisis point, a family member is quickly drafted to fill that enormous role. Often, the burden falls on a spouse, son, daughter or grandchild who becomes a solo caregiver almost overnight. By necessity, many families live like this for years—but the result can be exhausting and impoverishing. Sometimes, these heroic solo relationships thrive. Sometimes, they result in a downward spiral.

Especially with challenges as big as cancer, heart or kidney disease, dementia or major disabilities, even the most independent families are forced to widen their circle of helpers. That's why medical professionals, counselors and social workers all recommend forming a caring team ***even before*** a challenge arises and turns into a full-blown crisis.

A successful team spans a range of skills and commitments of assistance. Some team members may wind up providing daily service of some kind; others may only need to provide occasional help. Some may be hands-on; some may give their valuable assistance indirectly. Organizations like AARP use terms such as "caregiver" and "ally" to describe this wide spectrum of helpers.

In 2020, for example, AARP sent out a nationwide appeal for "service-minded public allies" to connect more broadly with regional networks of caregivers. AARP works with several other nationwide nonprofits in recruiting these public allies who are trained and then focus on many ways "to help create safe, walkable streets; age-friendly housing and transportation options; access to needed services; and opportunities for residents to participate in community life."

First steps in organizing your team

There are many issues families should consider when organizing a team. However, experts agree on several crucial starting points:

The person being cared for should be in charge. Obviously, some conditions may limit a person's ability to remain in charge—but, by default, the first priority of any caregiving team is ensuring that the person's wishes are paramount. That includes their cultural, ethnic and religious preferences. If dementia or some other chronic condition begins to limit that person's ability to make choices—the caring team still should try to honor preferences they have consistently expressed. This is one major reason that a caregiving team should be organized even before crises begin to arise.

Identify a coordinator. "Who's in charge here?" Veterans of family caregiving have heard that question more than once! Whatever term you prefer to use for a coordinator, your whole team should know who is in charge of resolving questions, organizing schedules and making decisions after family input. During intense periods of medical care or hospitalization, a coordinator makes sure that timely and accurate updates are shared with family and friends. That news includes whether in-person or virtual visits are welcome. During short-term rehab or long-term in-home caregiving, the coordinator is responsible for ensuring that all necessary roles are covered.

Agree on the smartest ways to communicate. One of the most common pitfalls involves the ways we choose to communicate. Someone gets left off a group email list and misses key information—or worse, a key event. Someone feels slighted because they don't use the form of social media that everyone else is using. Someone doesn't know how to check the team's online calendar. If communication turns out to be a chronic problem for your family, appoint a technology-savvy aide to the team whose role is helping everyone get connected. Sometimes this is as simple as showing someone how to load and use a free app on their phone. Read the chapter in this book about social media for further tips.

Expanding your team

Here are two valuable additions to your team that many families initially overlook:

Tell your supervisor at work. An AARP study in 2020 reports that only half of caregivers who are also employed have told their supervisors at work about the personal workload they are shouldering. Why don't half of all caregivers talk with their supervisors? Some don't have a good working relationship with their supervisor; some want their family issues to remain private; some fear such news might jeopardize their job. However, among the half who did tell their supervisors, most say they are pleased at the support they are finding at work. That includes practical programs many employers now provide to help in family crises. In recent years, more employers nationwide are developing services for employees and flexible work options to assist caregivers. Major corporations are discovering that these programs help build a healthy and reliable workforce. Remember: You won't discover what is available unless you discuss your situation with your supervisor or your company's human resources department.

Find occasional helpers. Start by looking through the other chapters in this book. Many of the most valuable team members may wind up playing only a limited or indirect role. For example, other chapters in this book focus on home safety. Who do you know who can assess your home's risks? Does your health system provide an occupational therapist who could visit your home and help with that process? Who can repair or remodel areas, such as doorways or bathtubs, to make them safer? Does someone in your family know a trusted carpenter or plumber? Add their contact information to your master list of allies. Bewildered by all the paperwork that is accumulating? Does your family know a trusted accountant, bookkeeper or financial advisor who can help? These skilled people may spend only a short time assisting the team, but their occasional roles can be very beneficial.

Caring for your caregivers

Here are some specific tips that veteran team members nationwide say will promote health and well-being:

Honesty and clarity are vital. Collaboration is easiest when the person at the heart of the team—the person everyone is working so hard to support—is able to clearly express their wishes. If they are physically unable to do that, then the coordinator needs to set the standard for appropriate openness and clarity. These values go a long way toward strengthening all the loyal relationships among allies. They play out every day in countless, small interactions. For example: Is your team's calendar of responsibilities easy for everyone to access and understand? Does everyone involved know about changes in routines? Does everyone understand potential risks and safety measures? Are questions quickly answered? Are changes quickly communicated?

Don't overbook or overpromise. A frequent source of avoidable stress is the frustration that builds when too much is packed into a single day—or when a responsible caregiver repeatedly fails to show up at an appointed time. Diminish the likelihood of such friction with proper pacing. Don't overbook the person who is at the core of all your efforts. Successful teams know how much this person is capable of handling in a single day. The idea of lining up multiple appointments in one day may seem convenient for the caregiver serving as driver—but that much activity may be beyond the capacity of the person being hurried from one location to another. In addition to proper pacing, talk honestly with team members about whether they really are able to keep the commitments they are making. An awareness of the team's overall capability is vital to confidently and reliably meeting a person's needs.

Reconciliation rejuvenates all of us. Good teams work hard. Good teams sometimes argue, even when everyone involved in a dispute has good intentions. We care so much that our emotions can flare. Forgiveness and reconciliation are practices at the core of successful teams. If this becomes a major flashpoint that you can't resolve, look for a counselor or moderator in your community.

Join support groups—plural. Many aging Americans already are part of support groups at the time a caregiving team forms around them. If so, encourage those connections to continue. But, remember: Support groups can help everyone in your team. Various members in your team may find specialized groups they can join for encouragement, tips and news that can help the whole team. What's their role? There's almost certainly a support network ready to help. Are they comfortable chauffeuring? There are groups that specialize in transportation. Are they monitoring a new diet? Nutrition groups are everywhere. In this era of virtual communities, support groups can be highly specialized. Are they caring for a veteran? Veterans' groups are ready to help. Suffering from a particular chronic ailment? Groups are ready to help, no matter how rare your condition may be. Have they found one particular support group to be unhelpful—or problematic? Find another one.

Remember: rotate, respite and rest. The best team coordinators assure that no one is called upon to do more than they can manage. Caregiving turns out to be an overwhelming, years-long commitment for millions of men and women. Almost without stopping to consider what lies ahead, a son or a granddaughter can dive into a seemingly endless list of demands. Every professional advising these teams encourages coordinators to look for ways to rotate responsibilities, provide occasional periods of respite, and get as much rest as possible.

Don't overlook distant caregivers. "I had to do this because I was closest." That's the story told by many heroic men and women and there is obvious truth in what they are saying. Proximity is required for hands-on service. However, don't overlook the many roles friends and family can play even if they physically reside far away. An accountant aunt in a distant state still could help sort out financial issues. An uncle who is a therapist can advise on treatments and can actively encourage a person—even through daily phone calls—to properly follow through with therapy. A whole host of distant helpers can send cards and letters, and initiate phone calls and video chats. Find ways to involve everyone who wants to help—no matter the physical distance.

Gratitude is gold. A growing body of research shows that gratitude is a powerful attitude—and can become a daily practice with long-lasting benefits to health and well-being. Gratitude in large and small expressions is a lifeline in caring teams. The vast majority of caregivers are unpaid. The work often is hard. Gratitude keeps millions of men and women going each day.

Caring for caregivers is covered in detail in a later chapter, which has even more resources for healthy, resilient living.

3

Our Assets

A realistic assessment of your wealth can spark fresh ideas

In populations around the world, wealth is a leading determinant of health and longevity. Wealth is your income, financial assets, physical possessions and the worth of other reliable ongoing assets such as insurance policies and pensions.

Yes, it's certainly true: Many poor people around the world lead long and happy lives; and, many wealthy people die prematurely. Overall, however, wealth is an important indicator of how populations will fare as they age. For example, the COVID-19 pandemic revealed the physical dangers of the wealth gap in the U.S. as mortality rates rose faster in poorer communities. As a result of the accompanying financial crisis in 2020, millions more families faced shortfalls in income and health care. It's important families are aware of the importance of a financial assessment as we age. We can't predict everything that will happen in life, but we can plan to make our assets last as long as possible.

That is why a planner, counselor or social worker is likely to start a discussion about healthy aging with questions about your wealth. Even suggesting this kind of conversation may be a scary idea, because millions of Americans have little or no savings and do not own major assets like a house. As uncomfortable as this kind of assessment may be, an honest and detailed conversation about your wealth—or lack of it—is the first step for planning how to thrive and enjoy life. The goal of this kind of assessment is not to embarrass anyone or to heap guilt on anyone's already sagging shoulders. The goal is to start building a list of constructive steps toward finding the resources you need, no matter what your financial standing may be.

In your own conversation with an adviser, there are lots of practical questions you may wind up exploring: So, you can't afford that second car or truck anymore? Maybe downsizing to a single vehicle— or going without a vehicle at all—will be a relief in many ways. Are you paying for a residence that is far bigger than you need? Perhaps moving into a smaller place in your community can cut that part of your monthly budget in half. Can't afford a membership at a fitness facility to maintain your health? There may be free or discounted options in your neighborhood, perhaps at a public pool or a fitness program run by a congregation or a nonprofit. These are just a few examples of the helpful and hopeful questions that can flow from a financial assessment.

Think of the evaluation of your assets not as a grim verdict about future limitations—but as the ground floor in building a new list of affordable resources you may be able to find in your community. You don't know what you're looking for until you know what you can—and can't—afford.

The aim of this process is finding a sustainable balance between our assets and the costs of our care. Aging at home may seem daunting at first, especially if you have to begin with expensive repairs or remodeling to cope with new conditions arising in your life. Then, you may need to enlist new caregivers or service providers. If you have to pay for all of these outside services, your monthly budget may swell by thousands of dollars. Lots of Americans find ways to avoid paying for such services by enlisting unpaid caregivers who often are family members or friends. Keep returning to the basic question: What should be our balance of assets and expenses? While some of our needs in aging can easily be met by unpaid helpers—others require paid professionals. Where should we spend our money?

If you are considering a move to an assisted living facility, you need to understand all the costs involved—including the impact on your overall wealth. There are many options. Perhaps you are living in an unsustainably large home right now. Possible solutions may include downsizing your residence or sharing your home with a friend or family member. You won't know your options until you clearly understand your assets versus your needs.

The overall goal of healthy aging in place is to avoid unnecessary placements in far more expensive facilities. That's partly because of the expense and partly because institutions like nursing homes may wind up isolating us from the larger community that has been our mainstay throughout life.

Who is most likely at risk of financial shortfalls as we age? A RAND Corporation research report lists at-risk groups as: single women, people with less than a high school diploma and individuals with long-term care expenses. However, the good news in that RAND study is that a majority of Americans will be able to fare comfortably as they age, largely thanks to the safety net of Social Security and Medicare to undergird accumulated family wealth.

Here's the most important message: Families don't know where they stand on this financial spectrum until they carefully assess their wealth and plan appropriate budgets. While millions of Americans do face severe financial limitations, most families can figure out a sustainable plan.

And, here's a very important reminder about this book: These chapters are designed to answer basic questions about the many issues we face as we age. In these pages, we are only answering the most common questions and providing widely accepted tips. The main message of this chapter is: All professionals agree that a crucial first step is getting a complete list of assets. Next, professionals urge families to plan for the future, drawing on either financial expertise within the family or by finding a qualified adviser.

That being said, each individual and each family is unique. Very quickly, your financial planning may extend into complex issues related to insurance, or to the values of your specific assets—or to a host of other details that may vary from one state to another and from one person's life experiences to another. For example, planning for the care of a retired teacher at the onset of dementia in Massachusetts will be different than planning for a disabled veteran with chronic substance abuse issues in California.

In this chapter are helpful suggestions as you start down this long and winding road.

Common recommendations

Here are some of the most common recommendations from professionals who work with families as they plan for healthy aging:

Recognize that financial questions may spark a difficult conversation. Family matriarchs and patriarchs may react with anxiety or even anger at the idea that someone is going to discuss their private financial choices. If that issue arises in your family, try to allow time and provide enough encouragement to allay those fears. But don't let initial avoidance turn into stonewalling. Don't give up. Anticipating and sympathetically accepting your family member's anxiety goes a long way toward easing the stress and making sure these conversations do take place.

Dig deep. Many families may be unaware—or may have forgotten about—assets that have accumulated throughout a lifetime. Examples of commonly overlooked assets: saving bonds tucked away "somewhere safe," a life insurance policy that may still have value, old-but-still-active savings accounts or IRAs from previous employers. Sometimes assets are overlooked because they are not immediately visible. Ask about a safety deposit box, a home safe or lockbox, a special drawer or an old shoebox where important records are tucked away. If you don't dig deep enough, a planner is handicapped in helping your family.

Don't forget the debts. Your wealth is your assets, minus your debts. It's easy to overlook or misstate our debts. For example, telling a planner, "Mom owns her home," isn't accurate if there actually is a remaining mortgage—or if Mom took out a sizeable home equity loan without mentioning it to the family. Without telling anyone, Dad may have maxed out a number of credit cards and paying back that high-interest debt needs to be a major priority in your new plan. Your debts may also include personal loans or financial promises that you plan to honor as you age. The best planning happens when all financial factors are laid on the table, including debts.

How to choose a financial advisor

In many families, the chief financial decision maker is the most knowledgeable and experienced person in the family—frequently a patriarch or matriarch who is used to making independent financial choices. Sometimes, another skilled and trusted family member gets involved. Financial decisions often are kept "in house" because families assume they cannot afford a certified financial planner (CFP), a designation that commonly is recommended by professionals. If your family plans to keep these choices in house, try to ensure that crucial decisions about assets are discussed among at least a couple of family members. They can provide valuable advice. Financial arrangements shrouded in privacy become a serious problem if the head of the family suddenly faces physical or mental limitations and, for the first time, needs a trusted person to act on their behalf. Even locating the records can turn into a crisis, if they are stored in a secret place—or are password-protected on a computer that can no longer be accessed.

Here are important tips—shared by a long list of financial institutions—about choosing an adviser:

Look for a certified financial planner (CFP). They are licensed and regulated. There are other kinds of certifications—as many as 100 different sets of initials that a planner may display after his or her name. However, experts writing for *The Wall Street Journal, Forbes* and other financial publications describe the CFP as a gold standard. Your family may select a planner with a different certification, but clearly understanding the professional standards of your advisor is a smart first step.

Where can you find an advisor? You could search online, you could walk into your bank and ask for help, you could contact a planner through an advertisement or you could ask a friend who already has an advisor. Wherever you collect names of planners, your best bet is to gather several names and then discuss them with informed friends and relatives. Keep drawing on the common sense of people you have trusted over many years. The choice is yours, but wise friends can help you steer a safe course and weed out the best choice from a list of names you have collected.

Look for the term "fiduciary." Financial-service professionals follow a number of different codes, depending on various kinds of work they do. The term "fiduciary" means that a professional follows a code of ethics that places the interests of clients first. There are other legitimate approaches to work in the financial industry. For example, some advisors have a personal stake in steering clients to specific financial programs. That's how these advisors make money and such an approach may be appropriate with clients who understand the risks and rewards of that kind of arrangement. However, most families who are trying to help an aging person facing significant challenges will want the security of an advisor who is obligated to prioritize the client's needs. That's why many experts favor choosing an adviser who is a "fiduciary."

Ask about payments. There are many specialties among financial planners, ranging from advisors who manage larger estates and are paid by taking an annual percentage of earnings from those holdings—to advisors who charge an hourly rate, or a one-time fee, to provide a list of services. Make sure you understand these arrangements before you make your choice. You may want an advisor who will set a package fee for developing a financial plan for your family. The National Association of Personal Financial Advisors (www.napfa. org/) is a leading network of fee-only advisors.

Financial advisors are different than accountants or stockbrokers. Need help filling out and filing your tax return? Confused about a particularly thorny account that you think is inaccurate? Want to buy or sell stocks? Other financial specialists typically handle those issues. When choosing an advisor, ask enough questions so you understand what this professional is going to help you accomplish.

Seek assistance from congregations, local nonprofits and community colleges. As in all of these steps, be careful. Predators can lurk even inside houses of worship, schools and community centers. However, in recent years, a growing number of congregations, schools and community-based nonprofits nationwide have begun offering either free or low-cost financial planning classes and seminars. Some of these programs are well-respected and effective. Even if you already have chosen your own advisor, you may want to attend a series of classes to beef up your confidence and awareness in the choices you are making. As always, ask trusted friends and relatives whether local seminars or classes seem legitimate.

Benefit from more than one opinion. Make sure to take some common sense steps before committing to a financial plan, especially involving significant changes in your assets. Take enough time to think through what you are doing. Don't make major life changes without fully considering them at least overnight—better yet, over a number of days. Family members may have wise advice to share, before you decide. You're in charge, of course, but making decisions carefully can avoid impulsive mistakes. Predators who target elderly people have a tougher time when someone stops them in their tracks and says, "I cannot even talk to you." That's because you've got your own trusted team to advise you. If you receive unsolicited financial advice through phone calls or emails, do not even reply. If predators persist, don't even try to engage—instead, report the attempts.

Use online help from trusted institutions, including the U.S. government. Most professional groups assisting families with healthy aging recommend the deep resources of the ACL (Administration for Community Living, part of the U.S. Department of Health and Human Services). A long list of planning resources can be found at the ACL's website (eldercare.acl.gov). That includes links to the National Eldercare Locator, a nationwide network that connects people with local resources. Another user-friendly website is www.medicare.gov that provides a clear and well-organized pathway to "get started with Medicare." There is a similarly user-friendly portal for Social Security at www.ssa.gov.

For more about legal arrangements that can assure a person's wishes are maintained throughout the aging process, even if major disabilities arise, see Chapter 18: Directing Our Care.

4

Our Gifts

All of us have strengths that give our lives meaning

We spent a long time writing and publishing this book for you, because we believe that each person has infinite value in our communities and around the world. Professionals call this a strengths-based approach to working with people. It's based both on ancient truths at the root of all the major world religions—and it's also part of a successful model that has proven its value in scientific studies of aging over the last several decades.

Quite simply: You may have serious problems now, but a person is not a problem. Each and every person has unique strengths, and has the human right to live as meaningful a life as possible. As we recognize this truth, our whole community becomes healthier and happier.

This might sound obvious, but entire ranks of public health and social work professionals marched into the early 20th century with some very different assumptions about dealing with the neediest among us. Sometimes, entire groups of people became associated with chronic problems. Sometimes, the goals of public policies were to control and even to combat entire groups of "problematic" people as if that was the way to alleviate suffering in the world.

Today, in the early 21st century, all of the helping professions now have long-established codes of ethics that, first and foremost, try to lift up the well-being of the people we serve. We start by recognizing the rights and the strengths of the men, women and children we work with each day.

Just as the previous chapter in this book was honest about naming wealth as one of the leading determinants of health—we now are sharing another equally important truth: Each person has both the right and the ability to lead a meaningful life. Every one of us has a unique array of strengths from which we can draw meaning and purpose to face each new day. And, that is good news, indeed!

Here are three universal questions we ask every day:

- Why should I climb out of bed in the morning?
- How can I make it through another challenging day?
- And, at the end of the day: What did I do today that really mattered?

These are echoes of the oldest questions raised in our religious traditions:

- Why am I here?
- How shall I live a good life?
- And: What is the ultimate purpose of the things that I do each day?

These kinds of questions—along with many others—are part of a strengths-based assessment. Before we share more questions, let's think about all people around us who have found meaningful work late in life.

Successful people who didn't debut until after 65

There are many milestones associated with turning 65, including retirement. However, a lot of people did not make their successful debut until they were 65—or much older.

Have you got a great story to tell? A long list of authors are publishing in their 70s, 80s and even 90s. Few authors of any age ever make it onto the national bestseller lists—but even modestly selling publications can entertain and inspire readers. Not every successful writer produces an entire book. Some popular writers post online stories or contribute to newsletters in their community or congregation. Love writing? Then, get writing!

The beloved American novelist Laura Ingalls Wilder did not expect much when she published her first volume, *Little House in the Big Woods*, in 1932. At the time, she was 65 and wanted to preserve her family stories. Her book found a receptive audience, so she kept going. She was 76 when she published her last book. She lived to age 90 and enjoyed some of the early success of her books. Today, her stories are favorites in millions of homes.

Frank McCourt's bestseller *Angela's Ashes* came out when he was 66—and he went on to win the Pulitzer Prize and wrote much more before he died at age 78 in 2009.

Peter Roget was a retired physician who struggled with depression and found that collecting and categorizing words lifted his spirits. He was 67 when he began to take this project seriously and was 73 when he published his famous *Thesaurus of English Words and Phrases*.

Edmond Hoyle was 70 when he turned his hobby of cards and parlor games into a series of small books that evolved into the worldwide standard reference on these subjects that continues to this day.

Duncan Hines was a traveling salesman. He had so much experience staying in hotels and eating in restaurants that in 1935, when he was 55, he and his wife, Florence, began writing about his experiences to help others find good spots as they traveled. They published a popular book. Duncan began writing for newspapers. He kept on traveling and writing. But Duncan Hines' real success didn't come until he was 73, when he sold his brand name to a national food company.

Not a writer? Perhaps you prefer the arts. Anna Mary Robertson Moses did not start painting until 76. She never thought that she had a talent for painting—but she was forced to switch from her beloved hobby of embroidering because arthritis prevented her from using her embroidery needles. Painting simply was easier as her hands became less functional. When she died in 1961 at 101, she had produced well over 3,000 paintings, some of which she sold for as little as $2. Today, now known as "Grandma" Moses, her folk paintings have resold at auction for more than $1 million each.

Love to tinker? George Weiss enjoyed tinkering with creative ideas in his basement even though none of his ideas proved to be a break-out success. He simply loved his hobby of dreaming up small-scale inventions and kept puttering at his workbench for half a century. Then, in his 80s, Weiss suddenly found himself the darling of business magazines, where he was featured in news stories about his invention of the fast-paced word game Dabble. The original game with letter tiles, packaged in a box, was so successful that, at age 84, he launched a popular Dabble app for smartphones.

Got a flare for the dramatic? Clara Peller was a manicurist, a very strong-willed woman who successfully raised her children as a single mother. She had already lived a meaningful life. Then, when she was 81, her talent as an actress was spotted and she debuted, in 1984, in a Wendy's commercial demanding: "Where's the beef?" Suddenly, she had a whole new career.

Are your talents in the kitchen? Harlan Sanders was a failure many times over and was all but broke at age 65. His first Social Security check helped to finance the launch of Kentucky Fried Chicken franchises. Although it was only a modest monthly income, Social Security allowed him to get into his car and drive around the country talking about his special recipe and cooking methods for Kentucky-style chicken. No one expected him to succeed. His life-long track record suggested that this was just another impossible dream. However, Sanders was right about one thing: His unique style of chicken was custom-made for mass production in the rapidly expanding fast food market. Customers loved the taste. He logged a lot of miles in his quest to sell his idea for non-hamburger franchises. To his surprise, his first franchise was in Utah—far from his home state of Kentucky.

Keep using your skills as you age

A major factor in success after age 65 is using the skills we learned and enjoyed earlier in life. That is especially true with athletes and anyone whose skills involve physical movement. Lots of farmers and ranchers are active well into their 80s and beyond. Champion calf roper Allan Johnson started competing in rodeos in 1946 and continued participating in his favorite roping event well into his 80s. Olga Kotelko, a Canadian woman who served as a torch carrier at the Vancouver Winter Olympics in 2010, held 30 world records and was studied by scientists because of her endurance. Olga was competing in sporting events, including the hammer throw and 100 meters, in her 90s. She competed in three track and field events the week before her death in 2014 at age 95.

At age 91, American Bernice Mary Bates was named the world's oldest, regularly scheduled yoga instructor. That record held until friends of Ida Herbert in Canada heard that news and Ida claimed the record, because she was still leading yoga classes at 95. Journalists believe there probably are even older active yoga and fitness teachers around the world. After all, the oldest judo instructor, Keiko Fukuda, continued teaching until she was 98.

Genda Guilfoyle kept professionally dancing in the chorus line of The Fabulous Palm Springs Follies in California into her late 70s. She was able to do that because she simply kept up her training regimen every week. Earlier in her career she had been a Radio City Rockette. She performed in 1955 at the opening of Disneyland in the Golden Horseshoe Revue. She never stopped dancing!

John Glenn was one of the first astronauts in the Mercury program and orbited the earth in 1962. He remained fit and, in 1998, he returned to outer space to become the oldest astronaut at age 77.

Sure, we might say: Glenn was able to do that because of the fame from his youth. His trip back into space was a publicity stunt. Maybe so—but that certainly wasn't the case with aviator Tom Lackey, who lived in the West Midlands of England. Tom didn't earn his first pilot's license until he was 80, a remarkable accomplishment on its own. He remained largely unknown until he discovered a truly death-defying hobby: wing walking. To raise money for charity—about $2 million overall—Tom would stand on the top wing of a biplane, tethered to the plane's guywires and buffeted by high winds for an entire flight. At 85, he wing-walked a flight across the English Channel. At 93, just to show he still had the stamina, he wing-walked through an

81-minute flight across the Irish Sea! When Tom died at age 96 in 2017, people across England mourned his passing.

The Guinness team has a long list of age-related records. As of 2014, the Hip Op-eration Crew in New Zealand was the world's oldest dance troupe with an average age of 79. Gisela Weser was named the oldest living professional dancing teacher at age 82. Johanna Quaas was named the oldest competitive gymnast after competing in the floor-and-beam category at an event in her home country of Italy at age 86.

Are those skills simply beyond you at this point? Remember: Everyone can do something, including working as a volunteer. Violet Robbins holds a world record as the oldest hospital volunteer—at 107. Think you can beat Violet's record? Then, get started as a volunteer right now and just keep going. There is an entire chapter in this book called Our Service with lots of ideas.

Popular jobs for people over 65

Volunteering is not the only option after 65.

Has someone discouraged you? Anyone older than 60 has heard someone say: "No one will hire you at your age."

If you are hearing that, you can confidently reply: "That's simply not true." In fact, a majority of Americans keep working after 65, although many jobs transition to part-time or are found in secondary careers.

Here are some of the most popular jobs listed by experts in post-65 employment.

Bookkeeping and accounting. If you already have this skill, just polish up your resume and look for a job. You're likely to find one. If you want to learn more about accounting and bookkeeping, afford-able courses are available in most communities. Some companies are willing to train new employees on using their software, because there is always a need for these kinds of financial professionals.

Part-time teaching, perhaps as adjunct faculty at a college or uni-versity. While tenure-track college teachers usually have master's or doctoral degrees, part-time instructors may be chosen based on your earlier career experience. Also check with local school districts, where teaching assistants often are needed.

Event planner. Some people are able to jump into this career based on their earlier experience in related work. There are affordable training courses in many communities, including certifications in event planning in some regions. You might want to specialize in one thematic area, such as weddings or corporate events. Some venues, corporations and even congregations employ part-time planners or regularly rehire planners who have staged successful events in the past.

Retail sales. Clothing, building goods, sporting goods, book and appliance stores all hire sales representatives, sometimes selecting over-65 workers because of their work ethic, their good relations with customers and their knowledge of the products. For example: Are you a retired builder, carpenter or plumber? Check out building stores. In addition to pay, there may also be commissions and employee discounts. Most grocery chains have over-65 employees. Some men and women over 65 jump into real estate sales because they have the flexibility and the personal skills to successfully start such a second career.

As you are starting a job search, look back over your life experiences. Were you a medical or dental professional? A nurse or dental hygienist? Working part time after 65 may be possible. Did your earlier career make you suitable as an office manager or administrative assistant? Do you enjoy caring for children? New childcare jobs are opening every month all across the country. Are you talented at needlework? Do you have the equipment and experience to do alterations or perhaps even tailoring? Your skills are in demand.

Enjoy driving and have a good record on the road? Many older Americans drive for a living, from school buses to long-haul trucks. Auto dealerships often employ safe, reliable drivers to help pick up and deliver their inventory of vehicles.

Questions that may help you uncover your gifts

Look around your area for free or affordable career counseling with a focus on over-65 men and women. You might find programs offered by a library, a local nonprofit, a community college or even a congregation. Training sessions may be available to learn about how to update your resume, how to effectively apply for jobs online and how to prepare for an in-person or virtual interview. You might also pick up good suggestions about employers in your region.

Talk to friends and relatives who are working after 65. Nationwide, the vast majority of job seekers now use both online resources—as well as word-of-mouth suggestions and referrals to find jobs.

Even before you choose a specific pathway to explore, remember that you need to keep asking those three timeless questions each day. We started this chapter with those questions. Here they are again:

- Why should I climb out of bed in the morning?
- How can I make it through another challenging day?
- And, at the end of the day: What did I do today that really mattered?

The natural aging process is likely to make those questions ever more demanding with each passing year. So, try to focus not just on your daily obligations but on your vocations—things you are happy to do in your life. That is why counselors are likely to ask questions like the ones in the following list. Consider asking a friend or relative—or a small group of people—to go through this list and talk about your answers. You don't have to ask every question on this list. Once you start down this path, you're also likely to think up your own strength-based questions to add.

What things do you enjoy doing?

What things can you do well?

What's working well in your life right now that you want to continue?

What are you proud of in your life?

What experiences have given your life special meaning?

What were you trained to do that you would like to keep doing?

Is there a specific part of your life's work that you would like to continue?

Is there something you did earlier in your life that you would like to return to doing, once again?

What was the most interesting work you ever did?

How do you deal with challenges that come up in your life?

When there's a problem, what are you especially good at doing to respond?

What are the most important relationships in your life?

What are the most important groups or organizations in your life?

What do friends and family say they enjoy about you?

Is there something a friend is doing that you would like to be able to do too?

What talents do you have that your friends and family say they appreciate?

What can you do easily that is difficult for others?

What do you like best in your community?

Is there a way you can take part in the life of your community?

What do you wish was different in your community?

Is there something you can do to improve your community?

What activities make you feel good?

What do you hope to get out of life?

What would you love to be doing if someone gave you the opportunity?

When you wake up in the morning and think about the day ahead of you, what are a couple of things that will make you happy?

What are you curious about?

What would you like to learn?

What makes you feel good?

5

Our Service

Using our unique talents to create meaningful change

Community service is at its core about giving of ourselves to address a pressing societal need. It is compassion in action. Through compassion, we connect at the deepest level to one another and can create meaningful change.

Volunteering in the community connects us to those outside our immediate social circle, broadening our contacts and world view, exposing us to new ideas and extending the reach of our efforts.

Volunteering also lets us use our unique talents, life experience, skills and passion to make a difference in enjoyable, life-affirming ways. It infuses our daily lives with purpose, meaning and joy. As Deepak Chopra puts it: "My soul expands when I help others."

For seniors, volunteering has been shown to improve physical health, mental health, cognitive function, and even extend life expectancy. It has also been proven to reduce isolation, a key issue as we age. In these ways, volunteering can serve as a lifeline not only for those we serve but also for ourselves.

In this chapter we take a closer look at how many seniors are volunteering, the benefits of community service for seniors, types of volunteer experiences and ideas to get you started.

Each year, millions of seniors volunteer. The most recent reports from the U.S. Bureau of Labor Statistics show more than 10 million people ages 55–64, and 11 million aged 65 and older, serve as volunteers. That's about a quarter of the population in those age groups regularly volunteering.

Why volunteer?

The primary reason we volunteer is to help others. Humans are hardwired to help others. It feels good to give and many of us naturally want to find a way to be of service. We may have watched our parents volunteer. We may have been volunteering since childhood. We may have deep convictions about an issue from personal experience or been moved by the suffering of a close friend, relative or group. One need only to turn on the evening news to see stories about food insecurity, educational disparities, child abuse, gun violence, global warming and public health crises. Invariably, we become aware that there is so much work to be done.

While we may set out to help others—volunteering helps us just as much as those we serve. Volunteering confers benefits at every age, whether it is learning a new skill or meeting new people, gaining confidence or broadening our horizons—whether we help one person or an entire city—when we give of ourselves, volunteering enriches our lives and lifts our spirits. Ultimately, one of the most surefire ways to feel good is—to do good!

Volunteering also promotes a sense of community, forging bonds due to shared values and commitments—and giving us a deeper appreciation of the struggles others face.

Many of these benefits are especially profound for older people. According to the Corporation for National & Community Service (CNCS), a growing body of research shows positive correlations between senior volunteers and their overall well-being. In particular, older volunteers experience:

- Lower mortality rates
- Lower rates of depression
- Fewer physical limitations/less disability
- Higher levels of well-being

Volunteering has also been shown to support:

- A healthy, active lifestyle (and in turn, improved health outcomes)
- Increased brain activity and preservation of cognitive function
- A sense of purpose.

What's behind those improvements? Here are just a few of the common experiences that raise our well-being:

- Increased physical activity (be it walking through a museum as a docent or teaching tai chi)
- Social activity (such as greeting visitors to a hospital or bonding with other volunteers while making care packages for a homeless shelter)
- Mental activity (e.g., balancing the books for your favorite charity or learning something new)
- Reducing isolation (which we describe throughout this book as one of the most common threats to our well-being as we age)

Best volunteer opportunities for seniors

There are countless opportunities to volunteer in every part of this country. The most popular forms of volunteering among seniors are:

- Collecting, serving, preparing or distributing food
- Fundraising or selling items to raise money
- Engaging in general labor, such as building homes or cleaning up parks
- Tutoring or teaching
- Mentoring youth
- Collecting, making or distributing clothing
- Contributing time and talent to your faith community

Whether you decide to plant an urban garden or deliver meals to homebound seniors, sew masks, canvas for a candidate or support the arts, volunteering enables you to improve our world. You can volunteer one-on-one as a tutor, mentor or senior companion. Or you may prefer to be part of a group that goes to a soup kitchen or to your state capitol to lobby. You may choose to use your expertise on the board of an organization whose mission aligns with your values and interests. In this capacity, you may plan community service opportunities, develop a new program, fundraise or help allocate funds. Even people with less mobility or a chronic health condition can make a difference from home by making calls, teaching an online seminar, doing web-based tasks like graphic design, or making blankets for people with cancer.

The most recent national data show that seniors who volunteered were most likely to get involved through a religious organization. The next common avenue for seniors was through an educational or youth service organization or another social or community service. A smaller set of seniors got involved in civic, political or professional organizations, as well as environmental and health organizations. Seniors also found ways to give back via sports and cultural organizations.

Who takes the first step? Most often, seniors take the first step by approaching an organization that interests them. However, invitations can be powerful. About a quarter of volunteers started when someone in the organization asked them to take a role. About 15% of seniors were invited to get involved by a friend, relative or co-worker.

Tips for getting started

No matter which door you enter, how you get in, or which form of community service you choose, let your interests, talents and especially your compassion guide you.

Before you jump in, ask yourself what you hope to accomplish by volunteering. For instance, do you want to:

- Improve your own neighborhood or perhaps a nearby, more impoverished one?
- Address a specific issue?
- Meet new people?
- Try something new?
- Do something meaningful with your spare time?
- Explore a new way of life and new places?

- Become more physically active?
- Use a specific skill or talent?
- Learn new skills?
- Spend time with a friend who is part of the group?
- Take on a leadership role?
- Feel good?
- Make a difference?

Thinking through these motivators can help you narrow down your search by matching your interests, personality and skills with a great cause for you. Read about local opportunities through the websites of these groups. Look at the organization's recent activities through their online calendar, newsletters and social media postings. If you aren't comfortable going online, ask a friend to help you do the research. Perhaps you will wind up volunteering together.

Here are some of the most common kinds of organizations looking for help:

- Food banks
- Places of worship
- Religious nonprofits that serve the community
- Hospitals
- Community youth centers
- Schools
- Homeless shelters
- Animal shelters
- Public parks
- Art museums, theaters and concert halls
- Youth sports
- Political parties and groups

Check out national organizations, too

Senior Corps is a network of national service programs for Americans 55 years and older, made up of various programs to improve lives and foster civic engagement. Senior Corps volunteers commit their time to address critical community needs, including academic tutoring and mentoring, elder care, disaster relief support and more. Stipends are available to enable low-income volunteers to participate.

Retired Senior Volunteer Program (RSVP) is one of the largest volunteer networks in the nation for people 55 and older. You can use the skills and talents you've learned over the years, or develop new ones while serving in a variety of volunteer activities within your community.

Foster Grandparents are role models, mentors and friends to children with exceptional needs. The program provides a way for volunteers age 55 and over to stay active by serving children and youth in their communities.

Senior Companions provide assistance and friendship to older adults who have difficulty with daily living tasks, such as shopping or paying bills. They help these adults remain independent in their homes instead of having to move to more costly institutional care. Senior Companions also offset the responsibilities that typically fall on family members or professional caregivers.

For more information, go to http://www.nationalservice.gov.

AARP

AARP offers the volunteer portal Create the Good (createthegood. aarp.org) to help connect you with a suitable project or organization. You can peruse the Volunteer Wizard on its website to match your interests with ways to give back. You can also fill out a volunteer interest form or search the Volunteer Opportunity Board (by interest, AARP program and zip code). There is also a volunteer helpline (1-866-740-7719).

AARP runs several of its own signature volunteer programs, including:

AARP Foundation Experience Corps connects students to caring adult volunteers age 50 and older who help at-risk children with reading and literacy. Studies of Experience Corps programs revealed student gains in personal responsibility, relationship skills and decision-making as well as reading improvements. Senior volunteers in these programs also showed gains in health and age-vulnerable brain function/activity.

AARP Foundation Tax-Aide offers free tax preparation to anyone, with special attention to older, low-income taxpayers. "Compassionate and friendly individuals" are sought to join their volunteer team. Roles include volunteer tax preparer, client facilitator, technology coordinator, communications coordinator, volunteer manager and administrative volunteer. Training and continued support are provided.

AARP Driver Safety Program includes Smart Driver, a refresher driving course specifically for drivers 50 and over. You can volunteer in this program in various capacities, including classroom instructor, recruitment, marketing, outreach and supervision.

In addition, AARP offers a variety of volunteer opportunities in the group's state offices.

National groups by cause

Google a cause that's close to your heart. For example, if you are or know a breast cancer survivor, searching "breast cancer volunteer organizations" may turn up a group such as the Komen Affiliate Network (komen.org), which enlists more than 75,000 volunteers in many capacities. You'll also find the American Cancer Association (cancer.org), which offers opportunities to fundraise, plan events, give one-on-one support to women with breast cancer, drive patients to appointments and advocate.

Most organizations have a specific link on their website to search for volunteer opportunities. They may also have a presence on Facebook. There are also volunteer websites that list opportunities sorted by your interest and location. One such website is idealist.org.

Interested in travel?

Many seniors look forward to traveling during their retirement. Now you can combine travel with doing good by volunteering with organizations such as:

International Volunteer HQ offers volunteer programs in more than 50 destinations, across 300+ projects for people with the skills and desire to help foreign communities in need. Thousands of their travelers are over 40, 50 and 60 years old and this program sees the wealth of experience and wisdom that comes with age as a plus. All that's required is a passion to travel and give back. Your skill set will also influence the choice of project. IVHQ offers projects suitable for those 50+ in childcare, teaching, language courses, sports, art and music, medical and health, wildlife and animal care, environment and conservation, community development, elderly care and special needs care, among others. You can take a volunteer vacation or do a longer service trip. Trips recommended for seniors include those to Peru-Cusco, Kenya, Romania, Morocco, Nepal, Costa Rica and New Zealand. For more information go to http://www.volunteerhq.org.

Peace Corps has engaged more than 230,000 Americans in its various initiatives to empower impoverished communities and promote health, economic development and food security around the globe. What you may not know is that Peace Corps is open to and actively recruits seniors who are "at a point in life where (they) are considering leaving the workforce, thinking about retirement, or excited to make a change—and a difference." Currently, seniors comprise less than 5% of the Peace Corps, yet are valued for their "special set of skills, wisdom and perspective." Seniors can use their professional skills to help a community learn about business or technology; teach in a classroom; or parlay their hobby into a youth development program. Some older Peace Corps volunteers find that they feel freer, are more adaptable and more open to others than when they were younger, and they value being able to lead full lives dedicated to social justice. One volunteer who joined the Peace Corps when she was 56 years old said it was "like having a second life." Another volunteer, a retired lawyer, said his age, 80, is a "definite advantage" because people in the country he serves "respect age" and he sees he can be "an active citizen involved in meaningful work." For more information, go to http://www.peacecorps.gov.

Advocacy

As gratifying as one-on-one or community-based, hands-on service can be—many volunteers prefer to make a difference in the world by directly shaping systemic, institutional, regulatory or community-wide reforms.

These volunteers may wind up having a broader impact on their communities by educating policymakers and other officials and creating a groundswell for change. For example, seniors can draft and collect signatures for petitions, volunteer on commissions and make calls to voters. Using what they have learned in either their professional or volunteer capacities, seniors can inform key policymakers about what is happening and what changes would be beneficial.

Many nonprofit organizations rely on volunteers to amplify their message and extend their influence. Some, like Habitat for Humanity, sponsor conferences during which attendees, including volunteers, learn how to effectively advocate and then meet with lawmakers on Capitol Hill.

Successful advocacy requires passion, preparedness and persistence. It entails relationship-building, vision and good communication skills—all skills most people acquire as they mature. To make your voice heard, see if an organization needs volunteers to do advocacy work—or start something on your own.

Community service for seniors is a win-win for all involved. The needs are great, the benefits are mutual, and there are many ways to get involved. What's more, each of us can make a difference. As Anne Frank once said, "How wonderful it is that nobody need wait a single moment before starting to improve the world." We need not wait to do our part. Find what inspires you and, with the tips and ideas of this chapter in mind, build your own community service legacy. Then watch your heart gladden and your soul expand!

6

Saging, Not Aging

A transcultural perspective on our gifts as we age

"It shall not be that time will leave its imprint on me—Rather, I shall leave my imprint on time."

That's an inspiring perspective on the gifts and challenges of aging, isn't it? These words sound like the wisdom of an American inventor or political leader, don't they? Perhaps Thomas Edison or Abraham Lincoln? You may be surprised to learn that they are lines from a courageous Iraqi woman who worked tirelessly as an educator, poet, journalist and human-rights activist before her life was cut short by Saddam Hussein in 1980. Amina Haydar al-Sadr, best known as Bint al-Huda, devoted her life to opening schools for girls, writing dozens of books and encouraging lifelong education.

Bint al-Huda's quote and her story are reminders of the need to expand our horizons as we age. A narrow perspective on the many problems that accompany the aging process will miss all the gifts we can discover around us, including all the wisdom we already have shared in Chapters 2 through 5. Now, in Chapter 6, we are further widening our vision of the possibilities of aging to embrace—well, the entire world. In American culture, aging often is regarded as a disorder to be avoided at all costs. However, in many of the cultures that circle our globe, aging is regarded with esteem and honor. In those communities, we don't become burdens as we age—we become the community's sages. That was the idea behind the worldwide appeal in 2007 by former South African President Nelson Mandela to form a global council of sages called The Elders.

When you see the word "transcultural" in the subtitle of this chapter, you may think right away of traditional definitions of "culture": ethnic or racial or nationalist or tribal groups around the world. But let's keep expanding our vision. What if the aging process itself is a global culture?

Consider for a moment: It is no surprise to any of us that we are all on a continuum of advancing in age from the moment that an ovum becomes a fertilized egg. This natural advancement into human development continues until our hearts stop beating and our last breath is taken. Regardless of when our last breath is taken, we are all in a forward movement on this continuum we call life. The stages of life mimic one another from beginning to end—assuming the person lives long enough to experience all of the aging stages of life. We begin as a fetus with a curved back, stand straight for years to come, then begin to arch into a bowed back once again.

As we grow, we have people who nurture, feed, clothe and transport us. As we age, we may experience that same cycle of life again. The difference is that the beginning of the spectrum has hope for a growing life that will be productive and successful. The end of the spectrum may proudly represent a life well lived—like a continually rising sun of wisdom and energy—but is often viewed, instead, as a burdensome setting sun. A deeper look into a transcultural lens may give us a different perspective.

Transcultural theory is not limited to studies of cross-cultural systems. Rather, the larger theory understands "culture" to refer to the unique life of an individual—or a collective group of people with a shared identity. Hence, we can talk about the culture of aging. Better yet, we can emphasize the need to see this process as a culture of saging.

The culture of saging varies from country to country, tradition to tradition, generation to generation and is also impacted by systems that act upon senior populations.

A transcultural approach suggests that we can conduct an assessment of our current lives by understanding how the following systems have influenced—and will continue to influence—each of us. These factors are taken from Dr. Madeleine Leininger's work as a nurse anthropologist and the development of her Sunrise Model to explain her Culture Care Theory that can be applied to any system. You can learn more about her work by visiting the Transcultural Nursing Society's website: tcns.org.

When we begin to see the world's aging population as its own unique system—a whole new realm of possibilities rises like the sun. Let us apply the model to ourselves and see if it's helpful to bring a deeper understanding of our current or future goals.

The Sunrise Model asks us to consider the following factors as we assess our lives:

- Educational factors
- Economic factors
- Political and legal factors
- Cultural values and lifeways
- Kinship and social factors
- Religious and philosophical factors
- Technological factors

These dimensions unfold in cultural and social contexts that are dynamic and continue to change throughout our lives. These factors can influence our daily patterns of living in healthy and hopeful ways. However, all too often, these systems wind up battling the folk systems we have inherited and the professional systems that emerge around us. So, the question becomes: How do we align these systems to encourage and enliven the best life possible? As we raise such questions, we begin to realize that the aging process is not merely an "ending." In fact, it is the unfolding of human life itself. This isn't a final problem to be feared and fought—it's a way of embracing the natural course of a meaningful life. As we age, this transcultural approach allows us to assess, plan, implement and evaluate the decisions we make, so that they align in the healthiest ways for each person, each family and each community.

Everyday factors to consider

Let's focus this theory on a real-life example: You. Here are some of the questions commonly asked as we apply this transcultural idea to family life.

Educational Factors: What educational factors are a part of who you are? As you age into a role as a sage, which educational experiences do you wish to maintain or strengthen? Where can you sign up for classes in your community? Do you learn best by reading, watching, doing or observing? Do you read on a Kindle, or prefer a book in your hands? Do you get your news from a newspaper or magazine that still is delivered in print, or do you get your news online or through TV? Do you like to travel to learn about new things? If you are challenged in vision or hearing, how can those deficits be managed to maintain your educational potential? Do you see an eye doctor often enough that your sight is as clear as possible? How about a hearing test?

> NOTE: *There are many other chapters in this book packed with more detailed ideas about these factors. To learn more about Educational Factors, for example, read Chapter 20: Enjoying Life. Consider this transcultural chapter a way to integrate all of these ideas we are sharing into a life plan that focuses on growth and empowerment and meaningful living with each passing year. Then, here are some of the other factors in this transcultural approach—*

Economic Factors: What economic factors will shape your life and define your choices for healthy living? For many more questions and tips, see Chapter 3: Our Assets.

Political and Legal Factors: What political and legal factors will influence your quality of life? Will Medicare cover your medications and hospital visits? Have you considered the legal tools that can ensure your wishes are respected as you age? In addition to Chapter 3, look at Chapter 18: Directing Our Care.

Cultural Values and Lifeways: What cultural values and lifeways are important to you? Do you wish to remain home—and "sage in place" with an intergenerational family system? Do you wish to keep driving until it's no longer safe to do so? Do you like to shop, golf, sing, read, dance, volunteer and use your skills to keep serving your family and community? How important is your independence and what does quality and quantity of life mean for you? How is all of this defined and communicated to others? Among other helpful chapters are Chapter 5: Our Service, and Chapter 11: Mobility Matters!

Kinship and Social Factors: Do we have friends, family—and extended family—who we wish to interact with throughout our lives? Are we connected with friends throughout the community? Do you belong to a fraternal, professional or social organization? As we age, we often have more time than ever before to build on these important relationships. As you think about this factor, look back at Chapter 1: You Are Not Alone.

Religious and Philosophical Factors: How are religion, or perhaps your own philosophy, woven into the fabric of your life? Is attending a place of worship important? Or, with whom are you most comfortable having a meaningful conversation about the meaning and purpose of life? Consider looking at Chapter 10: Connecting with a Congregation, and Chapter 21: Our Story, Our Legacy.

Technical Factors: As we live in a world of rapidly changing technology, what is comfortable and affordable for you? Millions of seniors now own smartphones, for example, but may not know how powerfully these little tools can connect us with the larger world. Look at Chapter 7: Going Online, for more ideas.

Glimpsing the far bigger picture

The central theme of this chapter is to lift ourselves way up beyond our immediate daily problems to glimpse the human aging process, around the world, as filled with potential. While the other chapters in this book answer many pragmatic questions—this chapter is a reminder to take time out to ponder the far bigger questions that men and women have been asking through the millennia.

- Who am I now?
- Who do I wish to be?

- What values are most important to me?
- How will those values continue to manifest in my life?
- How will I be respected and valued for the unique contribution I can make with my life?
- How do I want to be seen by others?
- How do I want to sage?

Are those questions overwhelming? Just as we encourage throughout this book, let's take this timeless wisdom and find ways to integrate it into our lives—right here, right now.

Take a pen to paper (or use your keyboard) and jot down answers to these questions. Don't worry about spelling or grammar or complete sentences. Begin to jot down words and phrases that respond to each of those prompts. As you write (or type)—and if you return to this list over time—you will be creating your own assessment of the culture of saging. Then, dare to share what you are writing with loved ones in a conversation about saging. As we write and talk and share and discuss with others, we are shaping our own destiny. Let's teach others how we wish to live—and they very likely will want to continue as a part of your personal journey.

Go back to the list of factors in the Sunrise Model. Which factors are most important to me? Which areas have I been ignoring—and now really need to develop? How can I repattern or restructure my life to embrace healthy saging?

The good news is: We can continue to be our own map makers—discovering new things about ourselves each day. Our lives are priceless treasure chests. Some of these gifts are obvious and only need to be shared in a more purposeful way. Some of our treasure chests are buried and need to be unearthed.

Let's aspire to be an open chest overflowing with gems of wisdom and knowledge we can freely share with those we love.

Remember the wisdom shared with us by poet Bint al-Huda? She wrote: "It shall not be that time will leave its imprint on me—rather I shall leave my imprint on time."

Unfortunately, in the Iraq ruled by Saddam Hussein, he considered her ideas—and her educational and social-justice activism—such a threat to his regime that she was killed in her early 40s. Considering the great wisdom about aging in her poetry, the irony is: She never reached what we think of as old age.

However, even in her youth, she followed the path of saging and gave her wisdom selflessly to the world, each day. Her words now have circled the globe. In this chapter, you have just received a gift from her. That truly is the priceless power of saging.

7

Going Online

Safely connecting with friends and family on social media

If you have a smartphone in your pocket, you are never alone.

Since the opening chapter of this book, our contributing writers have echoed the message: You are not alone. We all understand that isolation and exclusion are the greatest threats to health and well-being. That's why millions of Americans 65 and older are flocking to social media, especially since the birth of smartphones in 2007 and the explosion of Facebook. The majority of older Americans are online in some way, every week. Pew Research shows that more than 40% of Americans 65 and older are active specifically on the popular social media apps—with half of those preferring Facebook.

However, another Pew Research study reports that the "digital divide persists even as lower-income Americans make gains in tech adoption." The study found that 3-in-10 adults with household incomes below $30,000 a year (29%) don't own a smartphone. More than 4-in-10 don't have home broadband services (44%) or a traditional computer (46%). And, a majority of lower-income Americans (36%) are not tablet owners. When interacting on and discussing social media, it's important to keep in mind who may not be part of the conversation—and find ways to bridge the digital divide. That can include participating in community-based smartphone donation drives, setting up neighborhood internet cafes and supporting local trade-in programs for electronics.

These tools are a great way to connect with friends, family, community groups and congregations. But there also is a lot to learn about safely and effectively using online technology. First, it's important to avoid getting overwhelmed in order to enjoy your experience. Second, it's important to safeguard yourself from the occasional trolls and predators online. By adhering to a few straight-forward guidelines, you can easily keep in touch and keep up with loved ones while having a lot of fun!

Don't try to do it all

Friends are likely to ask: "Are you on Facebook?"

Or: "My kids send updates on Twitter. Are you on Twitter?"

Or: "I wish I could get stuff from my daughter on Instagram! Do you use Instagram?"

Soon, you are asking a tech-savvy friend to help you sort out all these options. When they sit down to discuss your choices, they might start by asking: "Are you already using any social media?"

You might find a medical professional, social worker or even a pastor asking that same question. All of their institutions, now, are on social media, too.

Those two words, "social media" refer to both the act of sharing personal media like text, photographs and video—and the platforms or apps that host this media, like Facebook, Instagram and Twitter. In trying to help you get connected, this person is asking whether you are experienced with any of these services.

Perhaps, so far, you've only shared with friends and family via email or text messages on your phone, which are great ways to keep in touch with people, but these methods are not usually called "social media."

If you decide to dive into social media apps, you will find family and friends telling you about many different apps they use. It's easy to be overwhelmed! Once again, remember: You are not alone. Even younger adults often find themselves deleting some of the apps that overload their phones. Everyone who is active on social media has found themselves overwhelmed at some point. Remember: You certainly don't have to juggle every social media app available for your phone!

Here's a simple tip: Start by asking the people closest to you what social media they use most often to share friendly photos, news, personal updates and questions. You don't have to sign up for all of them. Instead, select one app that is most likely to bring you the most updates you want to receive. Spend at least a couple of weeks learning how to enjoy the many options available to you from the app you have chosen. You may find yourself frustrated. You may need to ask for more help. However, once you are comfortable with it, you can easily add another app to your routine.

To guide you, here are short summaries of the kind of interactions you can expect to have on each platform:

Facebook: Friends and family can share text, images and video created by themselves or from other users as well as curate a list of friends who can see their media. Users can control who sees their content. Facebook also has a direct messaging feature that allows you to have private conversations with friends, family, acquaintances and even local businesses.

Instagram: Unlike Facebook, Instagram is primarily an image-sharing platform. One way to understand the difference is that Facebook Inc. owns Instagram, which it bought in 2012 because many users wanted to enjoy images and skip the rest of the Facebook-style options. On Instagram, anyone can share images and photographs accompanied by captions. While Instagram also has a private messaging system, it is a "publicly facing" platform, which means that users are encouraged to see posts from people they may not know. In other words, you're often connecting with the rest of the world on Instagram.

Twitter: This is another very popular publicly facing platform. Twitter is a way to speak to the world in very short texts, sometimes accompanied with an image or video. There are so many front-page news stories about famous people on Twitter that most Americans are familiar with it—including how easy it is to jump into other people's public Twitter feeds. You may want to use Twitter because you've heard that your favorite celebrities, TV shows or authors share their latest news on Twitter. That can be a fun experience. Keep in mind that all media and text shared on Twitter is public by default, though it can be made private by users who originally shared the content. So, Twitter is a very popular way to follow news about lots of people across the country, and even around the world—but is not an ideal place to share your most personal news and images with family members and close friends.

Goodreads: A unique platform, Goodreads is exclusively reserved for discussions about books and written media. Users can write posts and follow friends, but everything centers around books and book reviews. Goodreads is integrated with Amazon.com and Kindle to facilitate easy movement between those platforms. Do you love to read? You'll meet lots of other book lovers, including fans of your favorite books and authors, and maybe the authors themselves, on Goodreads.

These are just a few of the dozens of social media apps your friends may tell you they enjoy.

Once you've selected one or two platforms to keep in touch with family and friends, take it slow as you sign up and get used to the technology. Most of these services offer tutorials, usually including helpful videos. Spend some time looking around and familiarizing yourself with how other people use it before publishing your own media. Ask friends and family on the platform for tips.

A simple public-private test

Social media platforms have user-controlled settings that indicate whether a particular piece of media is visible to everyone. However, as you become comfortable with posting on a platform, take extra care to learn how to determine whether your post is public or not. Each platform has "Help" pages available to assist you.

Regardless of privacy settings, never post anything on social media you wouldn't want the wider world to see. Even if you think you are sharing an intimate photo or text with just a few close friends—those words and images can wind up circling the internet in an instant.

Here's a simple public-private test: Only share what you would be comfortable putting on a billboard that anyone can see.

Connecting with your community

When social media first began appearing more than a decade ago, it was primarily used to connect with family, friends and co-workers.

Today, social media can be used to make new friends and connections in online communities centered around common interests. Some platforms, like Goodreads, are based entirely around special interests. Others, like Facebook, have created or allow users to create specific online gathering places to discuss anything from gardening and small-engine repair to computer programming and baking.

These groups can be found by searching the name of your interest in the app's search area. When posting publicly or interacting with members of these groups, be polite, do not reveal personal information about yourself, and remember: Never post anything you wouldn't want displayed on a billboard.

Most of these special-interest connections are for fun, but many Americans with chronic conditions use social media for support, to get tips on valuable resources and to learn the latest news. There are online support communities for even the most specific disorder or chronic condition, no matter how rare they may be. The question is: How do you select from the many social media options that turn up in an online search? Many of these groups have become real lifelines to the participating men and women—but some groups that might turn up in a search are scams. A wise first step is: Ask your doctor's staff if they have suggestions about support groups. Ask trusted friends you have met through in-person support groups. Ask professional caregivers. Then, as you check out a new support group on social media—follow what is always the best practice online: Begin by listening and reading before you share yourself.

Safety tips for email and private messages

Email is usually not regarded as "social media"—but it is the single most popular way people use the internet to communicate. Close behind is text messaging and other private-messaging apps.

We often assume these are private communications, but remember that this information is stored by the company hosting the platform you're using. And, sometimes these systems are hacked. That means that you shouldn't divulge your most private information in case the platform's security is compromised.

Be very careful when opening and reading messages from people you don't know. Do not click on internet links or attachments from people you don't know, as they can contain computer viruses that will damage your device and put your personal information at risk.

If there is anything suspicious about a friend's or relative's message, do not click on any included internet links or attachments. The most infamous email scams can involve dramatic emails that suddenly announce your friend or relative needs help—and you need to send them cash. Where did such a predatory email originate? Your friend's account may have been stolen or hacked. Suspicious messages often look different than a friend's normal writing style, even if it looks like the message is coming from them. Compromised accounts may also send messages with unusual errors. If you believe your friend or relative's account has been compromised, do not even open the message. Instead, call them on the phone to let them know.

Never take any action online if you're asked to do so by a message from a stranger. That includes logging into a website, sending something by mail or divulging any information. If you receive a message asking for something and you believe that message is coming from a friend or relative, confirm with that friend or relative by calling them on the phone before taking any action online.

Never reveal your password through a private message. An authentic company's support staff will never ask you to type your password into an email or message. Any message requesting your password in plain text is a predatory attempt to acquire your private information.

Additional resources

For more information about enjoying social media safely, check out the following resources:

AARP runs a Scams & Fraud center that keeps you informed about the latest scams that you may run across online. Check out the center here: www.aarp.org/money/scams-fraud/

You can also follow AARP itself on social media! Check out the @ AARP accounts on Twitter and Facebook.

AARP regularly posts about social media through their blog network. To see their latest, check out: blog.aarp.org/tag/social-media

8

Caring for Our Caregivers

More than 50 million Americans devote their lives to our care

Millions of Americans 65 and older are unpaid caregivers for friends and loved ones. The American population of caregivers is booming! Even before the start of the 2020 pandemic, the number of caregivers nationwide had soared from about 40 million a decade ago to 53 million men and women. That's 1 in 5 Americans! According to a report from AARP and the National Alliance for Caregiving, nearly two-thirds of those caregivers are women. Millions of these caregivers are responsible for more than one person—and have suffered from financial and health problems as a result of their stressful work. The 2020 report concludes, "As the country continues to age, the need to support caregivers as the cornerstone of society will only become more and more important."

Overall, the majority of caregivers say they are committed to continuing this essential work. Most say that they feel good about caring for loved ones. Studies show that the majority of caregivers are positive about what they are doing, each day—even though millions of them took on these demanding responsibilities without fully realizing what kind of years-long commitment they were making.

The message of this chapter is: We all need to learn more about the stresses and strains of our millions of helpers—and find ways to support them. That is especially true because we know that millions of these caregivers continue to serve us, every day, even though they say their hearts are breaking.

That's a dramatic phrase, but it emphasizes the need to understand the deepest motivations—and stresses—that keep this enormous network of men and women working every day. There are two main ways that hearts can break. Our hearts can be shattered, torn apart into a thousand pieces that may result in anger, rage, depression and disengagement. But there is another option—our hearts can be *broken open*. When this happens, we may experience a greater capacity to hold on through all of the complexities and contradictions of our lives. This second kind of heart breaking can result in a restored spirit and renewed energy—an inspiring flow of vocational energy.

What is essential—and often overlooked in our families—is the need to talk openly and regularly about practices for the heart, mind and body that will enable caregivers to continue finding goodness and hope in life.

How do we get there? How do we prevent ourselves from *breaking down* in mind, body and spirit as we care for others? There are many resources to help us care for our bodies and minds. There are thousands of books about good diet, exercise and healthy living—from best-sellers about decluttering your home with Marie Kondo to cookbooks for healthy nutrition. But, before you purchase an armload of those books from your favorite bookseller, remember that there are deeper spiritual questions that caregivers must grapple with in whatever few minutes they find in their overbooked lives.

What role does spirituality play in a book about practical advice for aging? Let's start with the three most basic questions asked in a daily spiritual journey, as seen in an earlier chapter:

- Why should I climb out of bed in the morning?
- How can I make it through another tiring, exhausting, stressful day?
- And, at the end of the day, did anything I accomplish really matter—not for all of humankind, but for my small, task-driven world?

You know these questions. You have asked them yourself, haven't you?

Caregivers answer these questions each day through their extraordinary service to loved ones. The answers lie in the care of a beloved person—answered with hands, heart, lips, mind, eyes and soul. Through this daily service, many caregivers say, their own spirit is restored. Our challenge is to become aware of this daily spiritual, emotional and physical struggle that millions of men and women face to keep our loved ones alive. Our challenge is to understand that millions of our caregivers are not always able to maintain that positive sense of purpose. We need to build into our caregiving relationships times of respite and refreshment for these vital men and women.

We are talking here about all of us. Rosalynn Carter opens her excellent book for caregivers with the message, "There are only four kinds of people in this world:

- Those who have been caregivers
- Those who currently are caregivers
- Those who will be caregivers
- Those who will need caregivers."

The Family Caregiver Alliance defines a caregiver—sometimes called an informal caregiver—as an unpaid individual (for example, a spouse, partner, family member, friend or neighbor) involved in assisting others with activities of daily living and/or medical tasks. The people who are sometimes called "formal" or "professional" caregivers are paid staff providing care in one's home or in a care setting like a day care, residential facility or long-term care facility. Formal caregivers also may face the same stresses and strains as the 53 million "caregivers," but those unpaid providers lack the professional systems of support—including an income—that keep professionals going year after year.

Healthy support for caregiving depends on important truth: Every caregiver is unique. Every care receiver is unique. Every caregiver-and-care-receiver relationship is unique. All the stresses and successes, joys and sorrows, anxious and serene moments of those caregiver-receiver relationships are unique.

What is not unique is the basic necessity of each caregiver to maintain a healthy mind, body and spirit. The many strategies needed range from exercise to eating well, laughter to learning more about caregiving procedures, rest and respite. Entire books are devoted to these helpful strategies, including *Guide to Caregiving* by Benjamin Pratt. Major nonprofits like the Family Caregiver Alliance (FCA) offer online resources and training. The FCA's extensive (www. caregiver.org) website offers more than 100 free tip sheets and factual overviews of specific topics, plus dozens of free webinars—with new resources coming online every month.

It's important to start the process of looking for help before you or your caregiver reaches a crisis. As you get ready to dig into those resources, however, we can summarize some of the most basic truths found by millions of successful caregivers:

Think long and hard before quitting a job to become a caregiver. In countless cases, this quickly results in not just one person living in poverty—but two who now are impoverished. Caregivers should explore many options and ask for all the help they can muster before quitting their job to help their loved one.

Don't do the job alone. One failure of many novice caregivers is that their commitment leads to isolation with no attention to carrying a support system with them. To survive long-term, caregivers must find support from caring, informed, listening people.

Find a loving, life-supporting community. Caregivers benefit from looking for a community of people who will accept them as they are and will listen to them talk in an honest way about their life. This community may be a circle of old, dear friends. It may mean joining a support group, perhaps recommended by a medical professional, social worker or local nonprofit. It might involve connecting with a congregation.

Care for the body with good food, exercise and sleep. New caregivers often find themselves abandoning all three in their overwhelming orientation to their new world of service. Caregivers won't last long like that.

Pray, study, read, learn. As they all-too-often give up food, exercise and sleep, there is no time left for these vital ways that we nurture our minds, hearts and souls.

Sing, dance and write. Just as important is the need to express ourselves in whatever form we prefer. Play the piano. Sing along with the radio. Write poetry. Jot thoughts in a journal. Dance!

Laugh. If your caregiver is never laughing, it's a sign they need to pay closer attention to this list.

Practice gratitude on a daily basis. A growing body of research shows that gratitude is the driving force behind our willingness and ability to help others. What are you grateful for today?

9

Social Determinants of Health

We may have more assets around us than we realize

Our health depends on much more than medical procedures and pills.

Certainly, the many life-altering conditions associated with aging—including diabetes, heart disease, cancer and dementia—all require regular medical care. Then, as professionals develop a treatment plan with us, they will ask many other questions about what are called "social determinants of health." This idea stretches back thousands of years. In the Bible, Jesus says that we "do not live by bread alone." Many aspects of our daily lives contribute to our health and well-being. Since 2000, scientists around the world have devoted years of research to proving the value of these "social determinants."

If you hear that phrase while meeting with professionals, they are using that solid scientific evidence to look at all aspects of your life, your home, your family and your community to help you focus on issues that can be strong assets.

The U.S. Centers for Disease Control (CDC) defines social determinants of health as life-influencing resources, "such as food supply, housing, economic and social relationships, transportation, education and health care" that will affect the quality and length of life of people living in those communities. The long list also includes access to care and resources, insurance coverage, income and transportation.

In one government training program, a common conversation among professional caregivers goes like this:

"Why was Mrs. Jones admitted to the hospital?"

"Because the cut on her leg became badly infected."

"How did she cut her leg?"

"She was walking to the grocery store and a board broke on her front porch."

"How could that have happened?"

"Because her front porch was damaged in a storm several years ago and now some of the wood is rotten and her foot just went right through the porch, cutting her leg."

"Why didn't someone fix that porch?"

"Mrs. Jones lives with her disabled mother and neither of them are able to make a repair like that."

"Couldn't they hire someone to fix it with the insurance money?"

"Their income is so low that they let their homeowners insurance lapse."

"Who is caring for her mother, now?"

"She says a friend from her church is looking in on her."

"Then why is Mrs. Jones telling us she can't stay in the hospital? It looks like she needs at least another day or so of IV antibiotics and we need to carefully watch that leg so the infection doesn't spread."

"Because her mother requires too much care for the woman from her church to handle."

"Well, what is her mother going to do if we can't control that infection in Mrs. Jones' leg? And who is going to fix the hole in the porch? And, because Mrs. Jones never made it to the store that day, does her mother even have food to eat?"

This conversation seems almost hopeless, doesn't it? Poor Mrs. Jones and her mother are facing such an overwhelming list of challenges that they may be on the verge of a devastating spiral. The threats are very real. In this training scenario, they could easily wind up with two disabled people, rather than just one, trying to survive in a dilapidated house that seems to be crumbling around them.

But there also are assets in this story that the Jones family might build upon with the help of friends, neighbors and professionals. In the midst of their problems, did you notice their assets?

- Mrs. Jones made it to a hospital before her leg was so bad that it might have threatened her life. If she completes her treatment, she will be walking again, soon.
- They own their home, even if the front porch is dangerous right now.
- They live within walking distance of a grocery store, even if the shortest route is strewn with dangerous debris at the moment.
- They've got each other.
- And, they are active in a congregation. Even though the first friend Mrs. Jones called was not prepared to shoulder heavy-duty caregiving responsibilities, there are many other ways that congregation can help them.

Although it seems frustrating and even life-threatening when first presented to us, this conversation also reveals many ways that the Jones family could literally get Mrs. Jones back on her feet again—and these two women can keep enjoying their home and church. Identifying both threats and assets is the value at looking more broadly at the wider array of social determinants that impact us.

There now are many official lists of social determinants of health. Most public health systems in nations around the world have their own versions with slight adaptations for their regional systems and cultures.

In the U.S., the CDC's *Healthy People 2020* report lists these social determinants of health:

Economic Stability

- Employment
- Food Insecurity
- Housing Instability
- Poverty

Education

- Early Childhood Education and Development
- Enrollment in Higher Education
- High School Graduation
- Language and Literacy

Social and Community Context

- Civic Participation
- Discrimination
- Incarceration
- Social Cohesion

Health and Health Care

- Access to Health Care
- Access to Primary Care
- Health Literacy

Neighborhood and Built Environment

- Access to Foods that Support Healthy Eating Patterns
- Crime and Violence
- Environmental Conditions
- Quality of Housing

Those terms may sound cold and bureaucratic, but discussing these topics soon can point toward assets that are vital to millions of American families. Here's one common example: When talking about "social and community context" and "social cohesion," a key question might be: "Do you belong to a congregation?" Research shows that participating in a church, synagogue or mosque can provide a lot of social support, regular activity outside the home and a network of friends to reinforce the need to keep following healthy practices. It's certainly an asset for the Jones family.

Another crucial item on that list is "environmental conditions." Under that topic, a caregiver may ask about a whole host of issues that can threaten health and well-being, such as:

- Are there safe sidewalks and bike lanes near your home?
- How is your home designed? Are there built-in dangers that can be fixed?
- Are there toxic substances in your home? Or, in your neighborhood?
- Are there physical barriers in your neighborhood?
- Is there good lighting? Are there shade trees or benches where you walk?

When a helper starts asking you and your family lots of questions that seem to go far beyond your immediate health concern—they aren't being nosy.

They are truly concerned about your health because they know: Your well-being depends on far more than pills and procedures.

10

Connecting With
a Congregation

Joining a congregation is a healthy step

The vast majority of Americans tell pollsters every year that they are people of faith. In the U.S., more than two-thirds of us identify as Christian. One quarter of us identify as Jewish, Muslim, Buddhist, Hindu or say we don't have any particular religious affiliation. We are an overwhelmingly religious nation, compared with other countries around the world.

However, only about a third of us actually participate in worship services and other congregational activities on a regular basis. That means as many as 200 million Americans don't have a regular connection to a congregation—even though they think of themselves as religiously affiliated.

Now, research shows that taking a simple step—connecting with a congregation on a regular basis—is a powerful predictor of health and well-being in the U.S. and around the world.

Researchers in dozens of countries have been studying the role of religion in public health, especially since 2000. The Association of Religion Data Archives (ARDA), the scholarly nonprofit group that collects and shares such studies, has an ever-growing list of such findings, including:

- A study of older Mexican men and women over more than a decade showed a 19% reduction in risk of death, in any given time period, among those who participate at least once a week in religious activities. In this region, the majority in the study were Catholic, but the specific religious affiliation of the participants did not matter.

- Another study in Taiwan showed a similar pattern—religious attendance and private devotions lead to longer lives. In this region, most people practiced several Asian religious traditions, especially Buddhism and Taoism, and some were Christian. Their affiliation did not matter. Their attendance and regular religious practices did.

- A different kind of study in predominantly Catholic Ireland showed that regular participation in a congregation led to building larger social networks, which lessened the risk of poor mental health.

- In the U.S., researchers followed a group of more than 70,000 women for 20 years and found that frequent religious attendance was associated with a third lower risk of death, in any given period, compared with women who never participate in congregations. A majority of these women identified as Christian, but from a wide range of denominations. Again, the healthy principle was regular attendance, not any particular affiliation.

A 2020 ARDA report summarized many of these global studies and concluded, "Social and medical sciences are increasingly finding evidence to support how religion promotes better health, including living longer."

Why is religion healthy?

The authors of these studies collected by ARDA are scientific researchers, which means none of their studies have a religious bias. These scholars start by neutrally studying large populations of people, usually over a period of years. They look for experiences that predict a significant change in the participants' lives.

Around the world in studies that span the last 20 years, scientists have identified at least four religious experiences that encourage health and well-being. ARDA sums up these four in this way:

- You are not alone: Researchers studying loneliness are documenting the potential mental health dangers of a lack of human contact. They are finding that the vibrant social networks of religious communities offer members major health advantages, particularly for older people.
- Having a loving God by your side: Numerous studies find that an association between an image of God as just and merciful can provide benefits such as a good night's sleep, greater self-esteem, a lower likelihood of being anxious or depressed and having a greater sense of optimism and hope even while facing stressful situations.
- Prayer, worship, meditation and inner peace: Studies are strongly linking personal spiritual practices with health. For example, prayer can help reduce anxiety, provide calm and refresh us, especially as we face daily challenges.
- Promoting health through scripture and tradition: Most major faith traditions treat the body as a divine gift and preach against behaviors such as alcohol or drug abuse, gluttony and promiscuity. Highly religious individuals tend to take these teachings seriously, research shows. As a result, regular participation in the life of a congregation predicts fewer health risks.

Religious teachings on health

Christianity is only one of the world religions promoting healthy behavior. For example, healthy principles are a central part of Islam, which includes a ban on alcohol and encourages moderation in eating. "Second to faith, no one has ever been given a greater blessing than health" is one of nearly 130 prophetic sayings from Islam on health and medicine. For more than 1,000 years, Islam also has been known around the world for encouraging the work of doctors, scientists and other health professionals.

Each of the world's ancient religious traditions includes specific teachings about health and diet. Among other notable examples: Hinduism and Buddhism do not require a vegetarian diet, but many Hindus and Buddhists avoid eating meat. One of the Five Precepts of Buddhism is to refrain from intoxicants that cloud the mind. Many other religious traditions have similar bans on substances that can lead to an unhealthy lifestyle or addiction.

These global religions also have core teachings that emphasize caring for the well-being of the elderly, starting with the Ten Commandments: "Honor your father and your mother." One traditional Jewish commentary explains: "What constitutes honor? One must provide them with food and drink and clothing. One should bring them home and take them out, and provide them with all their needs cheerfully."

Healthy principles are associated with most of the major Protestant denominations that make up a majority of the U.S. population. Of course, many men and women who claim those affiliations ignore those teachings—but regular activity in a congregation increases the likelihood that members will follow healthy principles.

In fact, several denominations were founded along with core teachings about health care. Methodism's founder John Wesley encouraged physical exercise, became a vegetarian and wrote an early guide to home health care in the 1740s that was one of the first books on healthy living that thousands of early American families had ever seen. In the 1860s, Seventh Day Adventists were founded with health principles similar to Wesley's ideas— and researchers have found that active congregations of Adventists have significantly greater health and longevity.

No scientist is arguing that this is due to divine intervention or that one religious group is healthier than others. What scientists are saying is that religious communities have a powerful influence on active members' lives—and that entire congregations tend to encourage and reinforce healthy practices among members.

That is why the world's largest Christian denomination, the billion-member Roman Catholic Church, is actively partnering with the World Health Organization's special focus from 2020 until

2030 on a Decade of Healthy Aging. To kick off this decade, the Vatican hosted a global conference on Religion and Medical Ethics in December 2019. More than 250 religious leaders, health care experts and scholars from 35 countries met in Rome for the symposium. The conference focused on the healing impact of spirituality in two key areas: palliative care and the mental health of the elderly.

A report from the conference by Italian journalist Elisa Di Benedetto said, "This global movement of bringing interfaith and cross-cultural perspectives into health care systems has been growing in recent decades. That collaboration has been encouraged by public health experts around the world who increasingly point to the vital importance of an overall pattern of social determinants of health. This broader vision of public health acknowledges that a person's religious, cultural, social and community network is crucial to health and well-being."

Her report continued: "One of the great highlights of the Vat-ican-sponsored event was a call for an interfaith perspective in developing a holistic approach—considering both medical and spiritual needs—specifically in the area of medical ethics and the elderly. A very insightful panel discussion explored whether a coopera-tive interfaith approach could improve palliative care in communities where families come from diverse backgrounds."

For his part, Pope Francis preaches and teaches about the need for communities to plan for the care of aging men and women. In his many messages emphasizing this need, Pope Francis points out that providing this care benefits far more than the elderly recipients of assistance. Whenever he speaks to crowds of young people, Pope Francis says that their lives will be richer and happier if they spend time in relationships with older people—including caring for their needs.

The Pope likes to call young people the "bud and foliage" of the world's family tree, then he says, "but without roots they cannot bear fruit. The elderly are the roots."

In one of his talks to the world's youth, Pope Francis emphasized that any successful society cares for the needs of its oldest residents. He said to his young listeners: "You cannot carry all the elderly on your shoulders, but you can carry their dreams. Carry them forward with you, and they will do you much good."

This effort is more than charity, the Pope has said repeatedly. If young people allow a "throwaway culture" to dominate, they will lose the great wisdom of their elders. "If the young are called to open new doors—the elderly hold the keys."

Pope Francis concluded that all generations need each other to thrive: "There is no growth without roots and no flowering without new buds. There is never prophecy without memory, or memory without prophecy—and constant encounter."

11

Mobility Matters!

Should we stop driving? And, if we do—now what?

"You think I should stop driving!?!" Dad shouts. "No! I've been a safe driver all my life!"

That's a line from countless family fights about whether an aging person should hang up their car keys. Perhaps you've been part of such an argument. The CDC reports that this major milestone in life—deciding when to stop driving—is a part of more families' experiences each year as an ever-increasing number of Americans are driving well past 65 and into their 80s and 90s. The vast majority of those drivers plan to remain on the road as long as they possibly can.

This can be a life-and-death decision, the CDC reports. Every day across the U.S., about 20 older adults are killed in traffic accidents and 700 are injured in accidents. Thousands more are involved in accidents and other traffic mishaps that don't involve physical injuries—but may involve other very serious consequences.

We have twin goals as we work toward healthy aging in place:

- Safe driving (and not driving when it's unsafe)
- Then, remaining mobile even if we don't drive (or don't own a vehicle)

Let's start with an important question: Why do older drivers experience more challenges as they keep driving?

Among the challenges are:

- Slower reaction times—for many reasons, ranging from our physical and mental condition to the effects of medicines we may be taking each day. Even a chronic lack of sleep at night, which can develop as we age, will slow our reactions throughout the day.
- Decreasing ability to move our hands, heads, arms and legs quickly—from a wide range of conditions that could include arthritis, neuropathy or a general loss of muscle tone.
- Poor vision, especially if we are not up to date on our optical care.
- Poor hearing.
- Distractions, which of course can threaten drivers of all ages, but are particularly challenging for older drivers.

The U.S. Administration on Aging puts it this way: "People between ages 25 and 75 have relatively low crash involvement. After age 75, risk increases because motorists may have health conditions or take medications that negatively affect their driving abilities. Drivers may be unaware of these changes or unwilling to admit challenges to themselves or others, including family members. In the case of people with cognitive impairments, like dementia, they may be unable to recognize their poor performance."

Disabled parking permits

One of the most common adaptations for older drivers with disabilities does little to improve safety on the road—but can help a safe driver remain mobile by reducing the physical strain and falling hazards of getting to and from a vehicle. Reserved spaces for cars with a disabled parking permit were required across the U.S. in the 1990 Americans with Disabilities Act.

Federal law governs the policy. The permits typically are moveable "hang tags" or specially marked licenses plate screwed onto the vehicle. However, each state's policy varies on how these permits are provided.

- Permits are free in the majority of states across the U.S., but some states do charge for registration.

- Some permits are temporary; others are long-term.
- Some states have no expiration dates on long-term permits; most require renewals after a number of years.

Our advice is: Learn the rules in your state, so you don't get caught with an expired permit that can lead to significant fines.

Qualifying conditions also vary across the U.S. Only a few states recognize deafness as a qualification, for example. Many states recognize severe arthritis or lung disease—conditions that can make it difficult to walk longer distances. But you will want to ask your doctor, or your state's motor vehicle licensing authority, about the rules where you live. All states provide the information on their websites. Nearly all states also have informative toll-free telephone services.

Every year, reports of permit abuse crop up nationwide. On the other hand, many older Americans refuse to get the permits they need because they regard them as a public sign of weakness—or because they assume their disability is only temporary.

One common example is post-surgical recovery. If you are returning home from a stay at a hospital, your discharge instructions may include a referral to a professional—perhaps an occupational therapist—who can help analyze specific risks and adaptations as you return to driving. If appropriate, your doctor or therapist can ease your return to regular mobility by helping you to get a temporary parking permit.

If a permit is recommended by your health-care providers—take it! As we have repeated throughout this book: You are not alone. One quarter of Americans ages 65 to 74 are living with a disability, as are half of Americans over 75, the U.S. Census reports. Plus, the most common type of disability found by the U.S. Census involves the ability to walk—the main reason these permits were created. Do you qualify? Get one!

Drive safely

A parking permit only helps to avoid undue strain and injury while coming and going from your vehicle. The real challenge is the open road and the risks other drivers pose as you make your way through each day's travels.

So, here's some good news! Overall, older drivers try to follow safe driving practices more than other age groups. It's true! Although older drivers have more accidents, they do pay closer attention to wearing seatbelts, avoiding alcohol when driving and timing driving for the safest conditions. In other words, they are more likely to heed the advice in this chapter. It's a healthy starting point to discuss best practices—and a good gateway into a family discussion, at some point, about further limiting time behind the wheel. We all agree: We don't want to hurt ourselves or others.

Among the universal recommendations of safety experts:

- Always wear a seat belt and make sure everyone in your vehicle buckles up with you.
- Don't drink and drive, of course. But also, be aware of which medicines can make you sleepy. Talk to your doctor about coping with such medicines, such as taking them at night to lessen the effect on your response time.
- Choose the safest conditions. Poor weather and nighttime driving increase the likelihood of accidents involving older drivers.
- Avoid rush hour.
- Plan your route, if possible, to avoid congested intersections or tricky turns.
- Remain especially alert in parking lots where many dings, dents and non-injury accidents occur.
- Avoid distractions. This is a danger for all drivers, but multitasking gets even more difficult as we age. Don't try to juggle food and beverages. Of course, "hands on" cell phone use is forbidden—but don't assume you can safely use "hands free" phone options.
- Pay attention to the distance between you and the vehicle ahead of you. This can be a big challenge in high-volume traffic, but a proper distance gives you more of those precious seconds to respond to sudden stops.

- Dementia, including Alzheimer's, presents special challenges.
  You may be able to continue driving locally, even if you have
  been diagnosed, but you should talk to your doctor and
  family about smart limitations to ensure worry-free driving.

Consider this to be a learning opportunity. There are lots of free
resources for older drivers. You may be surprised at some of the techniques you can learn and adaptive equipment you can discover.

One popular gateway is http://roadsafeseniors.org, which is also
known as CHORUS (Clearinghouse for Older Road User Safety).
This resource is co-sponsored by the U.S. Department of Transportation. Spend some time on the CHORUS website and you'll discover
hundreds of columns, summaries of the latest research and driver
tips—plus links to other helpful websites. That information includes
advice on choosing a safer vehicle as you age and safety options
you might consider adding to make your vehicle more comfortable
and useful. Just one example: Vehicles with additional hand grips
and arm supports can make it easier to climb in and out. Similarly,
vehicles with easy-open locks, doors, hatches and compartments just
might extend the number of years you can devote to everything from
running your own errands to keeping up your role in that volunteer
transportation program you enjoy each week.

Another very helpful gateway is http://cdc.gov where you can
search for a free, downloadable brochure called "My Mobility Plan."
The four-page checklist is available in English and Spanish. The CDC
defines mobility for seniors as both driving and walking around your
home and neighborhood, so the brochure includes a page of tips for
improving safety at home.

Finally, one of the most widely recommended programs is the AARP
Smart Driver course, which you can find at www.aarpdriversafety.org.
This is a "refresher course specifically designed for drivers age 50 and
older." You'll find this program recommended by several state and
federal agencies as well as many nonprofits that work with seniors.
The course is not free, but it is affordable and is cheaper for AARP
members.

Warning signs

More good news: Millions of Americans drive safely every day well into their 90s.

However, here's the warning: All of us reach a point when we can no longer operate a vehicle. Perhaps our safe-driving adaptations will push that point until the final weeks of life. For many of us, though, that point will come earlier. The universal question is: When do we hang up our keys?

Here are the warning signs:

- Americans over 65 are more likely than the general population to get traffic tickets for failure to yield the right of way, running stop signs and improper turns. Have you received a ticket like that? More than one?
- Perhaps you haven't received a ticket, but ask yourself: Are other drivers honking their horns—or making rude gestures? Perhaps you're driving slower than the speed limit? Or straying out of your lane?
- Are you noticing new dents and dings in your vehicle, perhaps damage that you did not even notice at the time it happened?
- Do you get lost?
- Do people—perhaps on bicycles or at crosswalks—sometimes surprise you?
- Are family members beginning to talk about your driving in a worrisome way?

Having the talk

Perhaps you're such a self-aware reader of this book that you will avoid "the talk" with your family about ending your driving. You will know when it's time and stop without anyone having to point out the obvious need.

Most of us wind up in some version of the talk.

Remember: This is not only an emotional issue. It's a very important social determinant of health and well-being. If we can't drive ourselves, the discussion needs to immediately shift to how we will continue to get around. It's not merely a preference; a lack of mobility is a predictor of physical and mental decline.

Think about the talk in advance:

- It may turn confrontational, so make sure to allow plenty of time and expect a range of emotions in response.
- Try to avoid assessing blame for specific incidents, which can become a frustrating and circular argument.
- Focus on the safety of loved ones, including the aging person as well as family and friends who may be endangered by unsafe driving.
- Point out the potential cost saving of no longer driving—or no longer owning a car at all.
- From the start, focus on finding solutions for ongoing mobility. The goal of such a talk is ensuring safe and independent living.

What happens if the talk doesn't go as planned? What happens if a strong-willed parent absolutely refuses to give up the keys?

There are other interventions that can force the issue.

- Most states' motor vehicle licensing authorities have an option for reporting an at-risk driver and requesting that re-testing be required. Search your state's website for information on "older drivers" or "at-risk drivers." In some states, the person submitting a public safety report has to provide their name. In other states, like Michigan, this report can be made anonymously.
- Your doctor or other health care professional can be requested to conduct an intervention and driver re-test. Rules vary nationwide, but medical professionals generally can initiate this process, especially if they know a patient's history and have support from the patient's family.
- Your local police department may have to get involved in regard to safety concerns. Again, anyone submitting a report may have to give their name.

These options are too-rarely chosen by concerned families who allow stubborn and dangerous drivers to remain on the road, safety experts say. Most safety groups urge families to stand firm if the warning signs are mounting and the older driver simply will not stop.

When we can't drive

The mobility options across the U.S. are so numerous—with new nonprofit and for-profit options popping up each year—that it is beyond the scope of this chapter to detail what you'll find. But, let's be clear: If you stop driving—you must immediately find new ways to get around.

We should consider many options: One relative handles medical, dental and optical appointments. Share weekly rides to the store with a friend who enjoys shopping. A member of our church or club will pick up those dates. Most seniors have smartphones and can easily learn about mobility apps—for the occasional paid trip that doesn't fit anyone else's schedule. Is driving a burden on friends and family? As we age, if we give up our own vehicle, we save money and can redirect some of that to paying our share of driving expenses.

Contact your health insurance provider to inquire about covering the costs of some kinds of medical transportation. In addition, congregations may have vans or busses available to you. Municipalities and senior centers may also provide free or low-cost transportation.

Remember our main theme: You are not alone. About 9% of American households do not have a vehicle. That's about 30 million of us. The good news is that the majority of us who don't own cars live in urban areas where mass transit or other transportation options are available. The bad news is that millions of us live too far from the transportation grid to make easy use of public options. We may live in rural or suburban areas with limited access to any form of commercial transportation. If you find yourself in that situation, ask around your community. Networks of drivers can be found in nearly every community, if you know who to ask. From poor urban neighborhoods to distant farmlands where rural poverty leads to isolation, private drivers have been a fixture of American life for more than a century.

If there isn't some kind of mobility network near your home, consider starting one. If that sounds like a wildly impractical idea, check out the website (www.nadtc.org) run by the National Aging and Disability Transportation Center, which is co-sponsored by the National Association of Area Agencies on Aging and the Federal Transit Administration. The NADTC website is a great starting point for ideas about grassroots mobility.

Our message in this chapter is: If you suddenly stop driving or lose access to a vehicle, planning for your transportation is a social determinant of health. That means: Being able to get around on a regular basis is more than a personal preference. It's a predictor of health, longevity and well-being.

That means: mobility matters!

12

Home Safe Home

Making sure "home" equals "healthy"

Home is where the heart is, we like to say, but home also can become a lethal threat as we age. That is true—unless we continually update and adapt our homes with safety in mind.

There are many free or low-cost resources for analyzing the potential dangers in your home. Ask your regular health care provider. Many health systems provide newsletters, seminars and online tips about home safety for older Americans. If you are returning home from a stay at a hospital, your discharge instructions may include a referral to a professional—perhaps an occupational therapist—who can help you to find and prevent specific risks.

Falls and driving accidents (which are discussed in the previous chapter) are such major causes of injury and death in older Americans that the CDC combines both of those challenges in a free, four-page PDF called "My Mobility Plan." To download your own copy, go to the cdc.gov website and search for My Mobility Plan. You'll find a Spanish-language option, as well.

Let's start with a home-safety checklist. These risks and fixes are identified in safety guidebooks published by a wide range of agencies, nonprofits and even home-repair and insurance companies.

- **Rugs:** Want to prevent falls? Rugs are your biggest threat. At the top of nearly every home-safety list is identifying any rugs that can slide across the floor, trip a toe or tangle a cane or walker. This fix might be as simple as removing small rugs in

entryways, hallways and other rooms. You may also need to
remove or replace worn or fraying wall-to-wall carpeting.

- **Cords and other stuff on the floor:** For years, you've been
  able to nimbly avoid that tangle of electrical cords in the
  office—or weave past that stack of books or laundry baskets.
  Not anymore. The safest course is clearing the path and
  avoiding the risk.

- **More light:** Many studies have shown that plenty of light
  has health benefits, ranging from help with depression to a
  lessening of eye strain and headaches—to the security benefits
  of bright lights at the entryways to your home. Increase the
  wattage in existing lamps. Add more if you need them. You'll
  soon discover lots of benefits, including more easily spotting
  what you want to find—and avoid—as you navigate your
  home.

- **Stair safety:** Stairs are a falling hazard in most homes for
  adults and children of any age. Make sure your stairs are in
  good repair, any carpeting is secure and have stronger railings
  installed to improve your grip.

- **Don't fall in the bath:** All sorts of bathroom adaptations can
  reduce your risk of falling and may improve your enjoyment
  in bathing. If you can afford it, professionals can install
  walk-in baths and showers, strong grab bars and comfortable
  seats. If that's beyond your budget, a sturdy nonslip bathmat,
  shower chair and handheld shower wand are an inexpensive
  improvement. While you're at the store, don't forget a
  long-handle bath brush or sponge, often recommended by
  occupational therapists to help avoid too much twisting,
  turning and bending in the bath.

- **Tune up that toilet:** You may be astonished at all of the
  adaptive plumbing fixtures now available. Again, ask a
  professional to show you the whole range, if you can afford
  that. On a tight budget? You may discover that simply adding
  an inexpensive raised toilet seat gives you several inches of
  height that makes it much easier to sit and stand.

- **Wear the right gear:** We cover clothing in Chapter 15: Dress for Success, but home-safety guides always point out that many preventable falls are the result of footwear that slips or slides or flexes too much. Love those old rubber flip flops from the beach? They can trip you up faster than a loose throw rug. Prefer to walk around in your socks? Get some socks with grips on the soles.

- **Use the right tools:** Need to reach a top shelf? You need a solid ladder or step stool. Don't trust that you can easily balance yourself on a chair or the edge of a table or a kitchen counter—like you did in your 30s.

- **Ramps:** Once again, entire websites and booklets cover ramp construction techniques and regulations, which vary widely across the U.S. The most important advice is: consult an experienced professional. You and your family may find that a ramp suddenly is required to get you back inside your home after a hospital stay. Ask around your community about ramps you've seen that impress you with their style and sturdiness. Who built that ramp? You might need to contact that person sooner than you think.

This chapter is a brief introduction to the many ways your home can help or hurt you. This is such an important challenge for millions of Americans that AARP has published a whole series of full-scale books on home safety, adaptation, remodeling and repair. In fact, the U.S. Department of Health and Human Services' Administration for Community Living endorses these AARP books. Among the many guides, one valuable starting point can be found by visiting http:// aarp.org and then searching for "Home Fit Guide." (It's possible to get a free copy of the 36-page PDF from AARP.) You'll find dozens of detailed tips in that book.

Visitability

Does this chapter seem overwhelming? Each year, for example, more older Americans discover that they can't go home again—simply because they can't navigate their front or back stairs. In addition to all the other high-stress challenges in our families, we've got to find the money and the professionals to build a ramp. We find ourselves displaced or staying in temporary housing and, sometimes, we never go home again.

Since the 1980s, activists have been trying to change the mindset of architects, builders and homeowners nationwide with a movement that's known as "visitability." The National Council on Independent Living now hosts resources from the movement at http://visitability. org. In Chapter 14: Don't Throw That Away! we mention the way professional organizers have revolutionized the process of down-sizing. Top organizers like Marie Kondo have turned the problem on its head. Rather than focusing on what to throw away, Kondo recommends focusing on what we want to keep. Similarly, the vis-itability movement has recognized the overwhelming impediments that literally trip up families trying to adapt homes for their aging loved ones. Very quickly, families can find themselves neck deep in home-remodeling plans that they may not be able to afford.

The visitability movement says: Let's focus on just three things. Can people with common disabilities visit our home? Or, if we encounter disabilities ourselves, can we continue to live in our home? Those three most important things are:

- At least one zero-step entrance to the home.
- Doors with 32 inches of clear space to pass through with mobility devices.
- One bathroom on the main floor that someone in a wheelchair can navigate.

Depending on your condition and your home, that simplified list may be the starting point of renovations you may want to plan well before you need them. Remember: The visitability goals go both ways. You'll make it easier for loved ones with disabilities to visit you—then, if you need those adaptations yourself, your home is already welcoming your own return.

Enjoying home again

Let's take that visitability principle a step further. We have already covered the basics that therapists and home-safety experts list—but healthy aging in place involves far more than avoiding falls. Continuing to care for yourself and your home in healthy ways is a vital aspect of enjoying life. As we age, it's important to re-evaluate the ways we cook for ourselves, care for our gardens and outdoor spaces and do other household tasks, like mending clothes and doing a little bit of home repair.

In addition to helpful adaptive tools, families and caregivers should discuss any necessary changes to the home to ensure safety and ease of access. For example:

- Is the counter space in the kitchen accessible? Is there a nonslip mat in front of it to prevent falls and to cushion our legs and joints as we stand there preparing meals?
- Who will wash the dishes? Is there any easy way to clean up any associated spills, or do other kitchen appliances have to be moved to do so?
- Are cooking utensils like spatulas in an accessible place—and are they long and strong enough to use comfortably without exposing sleeves or hands to a hot stove?
- Is anything stored too high or too low for comfortable access?
- Have you ever warned a guest in the kitchen: "Don't open that because—" "Watch out when you—" "It's way back behind the—" Now is the time to heed those warnings yourself.

These checks can also apply to sewing rooms, gardening sheds and any location in the home that we frequently access while going about our day-to-day activities.

Once everything is safely squared away, consider finally taking the time to write down favorite family recipes you've always prepared from memory. You may find that friends and relatives will enjoy visiting your home if they know you plan to spend the afternoon making tasty desserts or entrees. If you have always been a talented cook, you might wind up offering seasonal lessons in how to make your signature dishes. If you've never been good in the kitchen, but now have time and interest in cooking, ask around about free local cooking courses. If you are part of a health care system, ask whether nutrition or cooking classes are offered as a free encouragement for healthy living.

Some of the best family memories are cooked up in the kitchen.

Home away from home

Notice that we are describing "home," not "house" or "apartment" or "condo." We're talking about your sphere of daily living, which could involve a wide array of housing. Beyond our doors, however, most of us enjoy "at home" activities around our neighborhood.

Here's just one common example: Have you decided to try bicycling for the first time as an enjoyable form of exercise? Consult your doctor, therapist or a knowledgeable sports equipment dealer about the ideal kind of equipment, including a helmet. A trainer can advise you on the best—and safest—local bike routes. A trainer also can advise you how to start this new activity so you build up to an enjoyable routine—and avoid overdoing it to the point you wind up abandoning the whole idea.

Staying safe in and around our homes should be our number one priority to make sure we can continue enjoying life for many long years. As we age, our bodies change and we have to pay closer attention to potential injuries associated with frailty and memory issues.

Take some time to discuss best practices with friends, family and caregivers, including:

- **Reminder signs and checklists.** Do you find yourself forgetting to lock the doors before you go to bed? Conspicuous signs placed in crossroads or on a bathroom or bedroom mirror in the home are a great way to remind ourselves of our to-dos.

- **Audio reminders.** Make sure your kettle makes a loud whistling noise when it's ready. In addition, extra-loud cooking timers will make sure nobody leaves the stove on.
- **Keeping a daily log, together.** Writing in the same journal is a wonderful way to deepen a relationship, and keeps the home running smoothly. Making a habit of writing down everything you need to remember later will help everyone feel comfortable and ready for the next day.
- **Deciding on check-in times.** It can be helpful to hear from a family member at the same time every day or week in order to build a healthy check-in habit. This is a great opportunity to talk about your day, as well as keep everyone on the same page. These check-ins don't need to be reserved exclusively for health or home-related issues. Have fun with it!

Taking a few precautions will set you up for success in and outside your home.

13

Emergency Preparedness

A 10-point safety list to help you sleep soundly

Many of us don't think about emergency preparedness until it's too late.

Do you know where the valve is for the main water shutoff in your house? Do you have an easy-to-grab kit ready that includes vital information and supplies if an emergency gave you only minutes to get out of your home? Do you have bottled drinking water on hand if tap water isn't safe to drink, which has happened in U.S. cities such as Toledo, Ohio, and Flint, Michigan? Do you have some cash in your home to tide you over if a massive power outage caused ATMs and credit cards to malfunction?

Are you prepared to be without electricity? To be without water? To be without essential services for days?

This chapter asks you to prepare ahead of time for the unexpected—from a power outage to a crippling weather event to a once-in-a-century pandemic. A little bit of forward thinking will help you and those who care for you deal with life's unexpected twists, reducing anxiety in stressful situations. The onset of the COVID-19 pandemic in 2020 illuminated the need for emergency planning, while compounding the challenges that seniors and their caregivers face.

Following some simple advice now will give comfort to you, your family and neighbors—even your pets—when events outside your control upend everyday routines.

A 10-point safety list to help you sleep better

Aging people can go through these lists with friends, family members and caregivers to make sure they are in good shape for emergencies when they arise.

1. Organize an emergency kit: The U.S. Federal Emergency Management Agency (FEMA) suggests making two kits—one for staying at home in event of a crippling weather event or other emergency and one to grab if you must depart your home immediately in case of disaster, emergency or evacuation order. Store these items in a watertight plastic bin and put the bin where you don't have to move lots of other stuff out of the way to retrieve it, such as the front door closet. As you prepare your kits, FEMA, encourages you to include:

- A minimum three-day supply of nonperishable food and bottled water
- Moist towelettes, garbage bags and plastic ties for personal sanitation
- Battery-powered or hand-crank radio, such as National Oceanic and Atmospheric Administration weather radio for tone alerts of changing weather patterns
- Wrench or pliers to turn off utilities
- Local maps if you can't access such on your cell phone
- Whistles to signal for help
- Underwear and a change of clothes
- Personal hygiene products, baby wipes and hand sanitizers
- Prescription drug supplies and copies of prescriptions
- In light of the pandemic outbreak, add face masks and disinfecting wipes to the kit
- Keep a stash of cash in the kit also, in case you don't have access to ATMs, working credit cards or banks that are open
- You also should consider preparing an emergency kit to be stashed in your car
- FEMA has other suggestions at www.ready.gov/kit

2. Pet preparedness: A basic supply kit for your animal companion should include:

- Food and water for at least five days for every pet
- Bowls and a hand can opener if using canned food
- A supply of any medications and medical records in a waterproof container
- Make sure there's a leash or harness available, and toys
- An animal carrier could ensure you and your pet stay together
- Consider how to care for the pet's waste by packing garbage bags or a cat litter box and scoop
- And put some photos of your pet in that water-tight container, so you can use them to find your friend if you become separated
- For more tips, visit www.humanesociety.org/resources/pet-disaster-preparedness

3. Cellphones and communications: Edit numbers in your cellphone to make sure key people are noted as ICE—In Case of Emergency—contacts. For example, include the notation ICE ahead of names of your children or doctor or caregiver: ICE Mary or ICE John or ICE Dr. Jones' office. These notations make it easy for a first responder or caregiver to search your phone contacts and find a person who can be called to assist. Cellphones may not always work in an emergency or natural disaster when cell phone towers may get overwhelmed. Keep a phone charger available in your car because that will help you during a power outage when electrical outlets aren't functioning in your house. It's one reason you may want to keep a landline phone in your home, even as more households move to relying solely on cellphones. Landline phones with a cord connecting the handset to a wall base generally function in a power outage. The National Center for Health Statistics found that most seniors still have a landline connection. In 2017, their study found that roughly 75 percent of seniors have retained landlines.

4. Want not for water: FEMA suggests storing water in containers for emergencies. At a minimum, FEMA suggests one gallon of water per person, per day. For a three-day supply, that's three gallons per person, minimum. That's enough to drink and to flush the toilet.

5. Label, label, label: Where are the water shutoffs in your home, including shutoffs for sinks and appliances? Label them and let every family member or caregiver know where they are located. Make sure they know where the electrical panel box is—usually in the basement—and label the switches so they know which one supplies light to the upstairs bedrooms or main floor kitchen. Consider labeling pipes in the basement, as well.

6. If you deal with disabilities: Contact your local police department to see if they keep lists of people with disabilities, so as to assist them quickly in emergencies or for evacuation orders. It's crucial to wear medical alert bracelets or tags to provide information to first responders about your condition. If you are dependent on electricity for home-use medical equipment, ask your doctor if there are alternatives that you can continue to use during a power outage. For more tips, visit www.ready.gov/collection/disabilities. If you have diabetes, the American Association of Clinical Endocrinologists suggests assembling an emergency diabetes kit, with tips listed here: www.empoweryourhealth.org/diabetes-disaster-plan3. If you require kidney dialysis, learn about what to do if you can't access your regular facility. If you have home dialysis, contact your local water department in advance so they can maintain a registry to restore service to you quickly, if necessary. Find out what extra dietary restrictions or precautions to take if disaster makes it impossible for you to receive immediate treatment. Other tips are available at www.kidney.org/atoz/content/disasterbrochurefacilities.

7. Let there be light: Keep a stash of batteries to power flashlights for every household member and caregiver. Do not rely on a cellphone flashlight for extended use. Put a mini flashlight in your purse. Beyond this, buy light sticks—such as those glow-stick necklaces that are a familiar sight at Halloween. The light sticks, available at home and hardware stores, can be bent to provide light for up to 12 hours. Keep a stash of matches around, too.

8. Copy vital documents: Make copies of medical records, insurance information, credit cards, prescriptions, wills, etc. and keep them in your emergency kit if you must quickly depart your home. Experts suggest keeping originals in a fireproof, waterproof container at your house, or in a bank security box. Keep important computer files on a USB drive for easy access.

9. Garage getaway: Do you remember how to get into your garage without using the automatic opener to lift the garage door? We're so accustomed to clicking it to get access to our vehicles. What if it fails? Do you or a caregiver know how to open it manually?

10. Prepare yourself and help your community: Does your city or township offer Community Emergency Response Team (CERT) training? Many do so, and for free. "The Community Emergency Response Team (CERT) program educates volunteers about disaster preparedness for the hazards that may impact their area and trains them in basic disaster response skills, such as fire safety, light search and rescue, team organization and disaster medical operations," says the FEMA website. The FEMA website offers more info and a CERT locator to see if training is available in your area. Visit www.ready. gov/CERT.

Want even more tips? There's a wealth of emergency preparedness advice online. Here are some other links to help you be prepared.

- FEMA offers many tips at www.ready.gov/plan
- AARP offers emergency planning advice, too: www.aarp.org/ caregiving/basics/info-2019/preparing-for-emergency.html

14

Don't Throw That Away!

Downsizing and the challenges of hoarding

Thanks to reality TV shows, everyone now knows the "h" word: hoarding. Our homes can become so overwhelmed with stuff that we can no longer navigate through our own hallways; emergency medical personnel face a nearly impossible task in reaching us through the debris; and, in extreme cases, floors and ceilings can crack or collapse.

If we are not compulsive savers ourselves, we may not appreciate the deep emotional ties many of our loved ones have to their possessions. In support groups for overcoming this psychological dependency, people describe their intense anxiety and sleepless nights over the possibility of losing their belongings. Someone else may enter their home and see obvious problems that seem relatively easy to clear away: heaps of old furniture, dusty boxes, stacks of empty jars, a mountain of old paint cans and ceiling-high towers of yellowing magazines. They see looming disaster and a potential quick fix—but, the loved one simply sees "home." They may be embarrassed and may have stopped inviting people to visit, but these mountains of material represent an essential part of life. That's why trying to remove their stuff feels like tearing down the walls of their home around them. This is not a personal quirk or mere stubbornness. Since the 2013 edition of the *Diagnostic and Statistical Manual of Mental Disorders*, published by the American Psychiatric Association, compulsive hoarding has been a recognized diagnosis. Experts tell us that the compulsion is hard to treat, often remains a heartbreaking problem for years—and the compulsion can run in families. More than 5 million Americans are likely suffering from this disorder.

Here's the good news: When it comes to the inevitable process of downsizing our lives, compulsive hoarding is the extreme. So, let's turn this chapter, now, to the universal challenge of simply downsizing. The vast majority of us are not hoarders. However, like our earlier chapter on driving—everyone downsizes in the end. Some of us try to keep every scrap we own until our dying day, but none of us can take it with us after that. So, every year, millions of us downsize.

Downsizing our homes

Throughout this book, we have recommended many resources produced by AARP. In Chapter 12: Home Safe Home, we pointed out the many short AARP publications on home safety, repair and adaptation for disabilities. When it comes to downsizing, AARP experts recognized the enormous, complex challenges all families face—so the AARP standard reference book on downsizing is 256 pages. It's available on the aarp.org website, as well as Amazon.com and other online booksellers. Look for *Downsizing the Family Home: What to Save, What to Let Go* by Marni Jameson. You may recognize her name, because she is a popular journalist who writes about home management for major newspapers and magazines. The book she produced for AARP is exhaustive in covering every nook and cranny of this issue.

Of course, there are also hundreds of other valuable guides to this process—from free brochures and booklets to full-scale books and even interactive workbooks. Currently, one of the leading names in downsizing is Marie Kondo. Visit her konmari.com website. She is the author of several best-selling books.

Kondo is the latest star in the ever-expanding movement called "professional organizing." In the U.S., one of the leading organizations promoting best practices in this emerging field is the Institute for Challenging Disorganization. Their website is www.challengingdisorganization.org/. Most importantly, you can enter your zip code to find names of organizers in your area. The website includes a code of ethics under the "About Us" link. Those principles reflect the worldwide efforts of the International Federation of Professional Organizing Associations, which was founded in 2006 in Canada.

Why is it important to carefully check out consultants before engaging one? This business is booming and there are countless services you can find on Google that come with hefty price tags. While the groups we just mentioned are trying to hold service providers to higher standards of training and operation, the multi-billion-dollar home organization market remains a Wild West of competing offers. We recommend starting with some inexpensive research, which might include ordering a book by AARP or Kondo. Get a feel for the challenges you are facing—and your family goals. Then, if you need a professional consultant, carefully check your local options.

Whether you wind up making your own plan, following a guidebook, or hiring a consultant—the overall goal should be to improve health, well-being and the enjoyment of life. That's the reason so many people have flocked to the books and TV shows featuring consultants like Marie Kondo. Her strategy—and the approach of others like her—turns this enormous challenge on its head. If an individual, or an entire family, decides to downsize, we tend to start with the biggest problem areas. We want to clear out the garage, the attic, the basement or the overflowing closets. We dive into the deepest mess—and may not emerge for many months. Instead, Kondo and others suggest we begin by focusing on the smaller number of items that are absolute essentials in our lives. Kondo's famous test is: "What sparks joy?" Rather than obsessing over each item we may have to give up—we focus on the short list of items that truly make life worth living. In her books and TV series, she also describes these essentials as "things close to your heart." She distinguishes those from possessions we want to save—because "we might need them." That second category often is the rationale for hoarding.

Where should we begin?

As we have just seen, organizers vary widely in the methods they recommend. An approach similar to the Kondo method might begin with clothing. We gather all of our clothing from every part of our home into a single sorting area. Next, a carefully selected pile is set aside to save. The rest is donated to appropriate charities or community groups, depending on the condition and value of the clothing. After that, another category is chosen: perhaps books or recordings or tools or recreational items.

However, many downsizing experts argue that families may not have enough time and energy to pursue a more elaborate method that could take months to complete. So, an alternative starting point is summed up in two words: Think big!

A think-big approach starts with the question: What are the largest objects cluttering your home? Usually they are vehicles. Look back at Chapter 11: Mobility Matters! Perhaps this is a time to make do with a single car—or to quit driving altogether. Giving up our vehicles is a major decision that raises other questions, such as: How will we remain mobile? On the other hand, getting rid of our vehicles—perhaps by selling them or donating them to charity—is a quick way to open up space around a home. Even if we need to keep our primary vehicle, getting rid of second or third vehicles will be a big cost-saving move by eliminating licensing fees, insurance costs and ongoing repair bills for those aging cars.

Advocates of the think-big approach also urge families to look for:

- Anything you've placed in off-site storage, which has become another multi-billion-dollar business across the U.S. Simply the fact that you have stored these things away from your home usually means that they are not essentials. Ending those monthly rental fees also helps the family budget. Donations could provide tax advantages.

- Broken appliances, including washers and dryers and TVs that were stored because "we might need them" for some reason in the future.

- Unused appliances. If you haven't used an appliance in the past year, you're unlikely to need it in the future. While it's true that many power tools and appliances are seasonal essentials, including snow blowers and lawn mowers, the haven't-used-it-in-a-year test can quickly identify those big items you can donate, recycle or discard.

- Exercise equipment you haven't used in a year—especially if that equipment is broken or in poor repair. This often is an especially painful choice, because keeping fit is essential as we age. The best way to make these decisions is to be honest about your own fitness plan—and then be honest about whether you will use devices you are storing. Perhaps your equipment is no longer appropriate to your range of motion. Perhaps your device is broken. Millions of homes are heaped with outdated or unusable equipment that "just needs to be fixed." Even if the equipment still works, ask yourself: Can I even see it anymore? Have I turned it into a clothing rack?

- Furniture in "spare rooms" or "guest rooms." This often seems like a convenient strategy for parking family furniture— dressers, chairs, desks, beds, bookshelves—with the good intention that we are saving them for family and friends to use. Often, getting rid of these big items—starting with spare dressers and unused desks—represent a great way to kick-start your downsizing. Especially if this furniture is in good repair, you'll likely find family, friends, charities or local nonprofits who will be thrilled to receive these gifts. There might even be a tax benefit.

- "Antiques." We put that term in quotes because tons of old furniture, tools, musical instruments, appliances, framed objects and knickknacks are gathering dust in our homes because these things are old and we assume they have value. We have all seen TV shows in which someone's dusty knickknack turns out to be worth a great deal of money. However, in most cases—our stuff is merely old. If you think you own valuable antiques, ask a professional to look over these objects. Each year, families discover that they have to wind up paying people to remove heavy objects, like that century-old piano in the living room that hasn't been tuned in ages.

Here are some of the other starting points organizers identify in downsizing:

- Classic magazines. Americans just hate to toss old issues of National Geographic, for example. Structural engineers rank old magazines and newspapers as one of the greatest threats to the rafters in many homes.

- Extra dishes, tableware, glasses and mugs. Sure, you got that coffee mug at Niagara Falls, and that heavy box of dishes once belonged to your aunt, but your fond family memories don't depend on those heavy cartons remaining in your closet or basement. Unlike old magazines, many nonprofits across the U.S. will take complete, unbroken sets of dishes and tableware.

- Greeting cards and holiday decorations. Some family homes have surprisingly large piles of greeting cards—including boxes of unused cards—as well as holiday decorations. Americans spend billions of dollars each year on ornamenting their homes for New Year's, Easter, Halloween, Thanksgiving and Christmas. What to toss or recycle? Recall that handy haven't-used-it-in-a-year test? If you haven't hauled out that 6-foot-tall plastic snowman and you haven't strung those 500 lights along the rafters for more than a year—you're unlikely to use them in the future.

- Luggage. Most of us have accumulated more luggage than we need. For each person living in the home, keep a bag that is sturdy, convenient, ample for most trips and easy to wheel around. Get rid of the rest. That includes all the dusty pet carriers and cages in the garage or basement.

- Home repair or crafting leftovers. Far too many homes are jammed with extra pieces of wood, old windows, heaps of extra shingles, tool kits we only used once, cans of paints or sealants, plastic bins full of yarn or scrapbooking supplies— the list goes on and on. Why have we kept this stuff in the first place? This is the classic case of avoidance with the excuse: "We might need that someday." In truth: No, we won't.

- Out-of-date stockpiles of cans and boxes of food. Usually, a startling amount of room can be made in kitchens, closets and pantries by simply getting rid of all the out-of-date boxes of cereal, sacks of flour, canned goods and bottles of sauces and condiments. If this is a challenge in your family, you might even turn this into a game. Who can find the oldest product in the kitchen cabinets? And don't forget to look in the back of the refrigerator and the bottom of the freezer.

- Stuff your kids left with you. One of the joys of aging is reaching the point when you can call your kids and say: "Pay me a visit and sort out the stuff you want to take with you—because the rest is being donated to charity." If you do this right, you may wind up planning a delightful visit filled with lots of laughter and warm memories. But, be strict. Set a date. Our kids are as prone to delay downsizing as we are.

When do we need help?

In some households, compulsive hoarding dashes these optimistic plans and turns downsizing into a nightmare. Our advice is: If hoarding has become a deeply entrenched pattern in your family, you will need to summon lots of time, compassion and kindness.

Ever since compulsive hoarding became an officially recognized diagnosis, professional researchers have looked for solutions. As of this writing, there is no medication specifically approved for treating this disorder. Talking with a counselor, therapist or psychologist may help. If there is a local support group in your community—and these groups are expanding each year—then you may find some assistance there. However, the professional consensus is that this chronic condition is not easy to resolve and usually continues to worsen as we age. Despite your best efforts to confront this challenge in your family, you may not succeed.

What signs should we look for to identify an emerging problem?

- Hoarding tends to run in families.
- Recent research indicates that a tendency toward hoarding can be identified even in young adults.

- Trauma or other stressful periods in one's life can contribute
  to the problem, leading to a fear of getting rid of anything
  that might be needed to cope with a future crisis.
- The condition may be associated with other health challenges,
  such as chronic depression and anxiety or alcohol dependence.
- Researchers distinguish hoarding from obsessive-compulsive
  disorder, however, the two conditions are related in many
  cases.

Hoarding gets progressively worse. So, intervening as early as
possible is advised. Look for:

- An unwillingness to recycle or throw away newspapers,
  magazines and junk mail.
- Storing broken appliances.
- Kitchen cupboards or refrigerators that are too full to hold
  new groceries.
- Kitchen counters that are too full to use them for food
  preparation.
- Bathroom fixtures like tubs or showers that are used for
  storage.
- A reluctance to let people visit because "the house is a mess."
- Living with more cats or dogs than can be cared for properly.

That's serious stuff in many families. But, let's end this chapter with
some good news. As we said at the start, the majority of Americans
are not hoarders. As a result, in millions of households, downsizing can become a joyous opportunity for family reunions. Over a
number of weeks or months, far-flung family members and friends
may pay visits to help with the process. Fond memories can resurface.
Everyone can feel good about making donations to community
groups. Old photos, letters, recipes and other keepsakes are handed
along to the next generation.

Downsizing can become a true gift as we age.

15

Dress for Success

Feeling confident helps to build 'social capital'

We all have a right to feel good about ourselves, no matter our age or physical condition.

There is strong evidence that personal confidence contributes to what professionals call our "social capital," our ability to form relationships that improve our overall well-being. It's hard to feel confident if we don't like how we look—or if our clothing constricts our movement. One important way we build that confidence—and our sense of independence—is through our clothing and the handy gear we carry with us. As we age, that can become a real challenge. We may have medical conditions that limit our mobility, or we may have a medical diagnosis that has left us with limited functions due to a stroke, arthritis, dementia, diabetes or some other chronic condition.

The message of this chapter is simple: Part of healthy living includes paying attention to what we wear and carry with us on a daily basis.

Yes, we know that some readers will want to highlight that last sentence in a bright color—so they can show it to family and friends to explain why they want to spend a little more time, and perhaps a bit more money, on appearance and gear.

You can say: "This isn't vanity! It's good for my health!"

Movement and mobility

Let's start with movement and mobility. If you have limitations, you will need to assess whether you are able to dress independently—or need help. You will need to consider whether you will be regularly using a wheelchair or a walker. Talk to your doctor or therapist about the likely progression of your condition. What's likely to happen over the next year? This is important to consider when organizing your closet.

An AARP report on healthy aging strongly emphasizes this priority: "While no two caretakers face the same day-to-day issues, one universal strain remains: the inherent challenge of dressing loved ones who can't dress themselves." The AARP report says that struggles over clothing are an all-too-common flash point "and can be the breaking point for families." That's because it's such a daily, intimate experience, the report says.

This chapter is not an exhaustive list of your options. You can find entire catalogues—both printed catalogues and online listings—that detail thousands of choices. Our purpose in this chapter is to emphasize to you and your family the importance of carefully planning what you'll wear and carry.

Adaptive clothing

Adaptive clothing can be ordered online, or you can adapt your current wardrobe to meet your needs. And, as you buy new outfits or adapt your old ones, remember our main message: You have the right to look good and feel confident! For many older Americans, adapting favorite outfits might be a creative task that someone in your family is able to do for you. If not, ask around in your community. There are many women and men who do alterations and tailoring on the side. Some nonprofits have sewing auxiliaries.

What adaptations are needed? Please consult with medical personnel, therapists or caregivers about specific questions involving clothing. Here are some of the most common issues to ask about and consider:

- Add pockets for convenient storage of daily necessities.
- Choose soft fabrics to avoid irritation of sensitive, thinning skin.
- Avoid seams that can cause pressure spots. Do you like denim? Then, you may want to avoid those especially rough denim seams. Look for seamless denim garments.
- Replace drawstrings in clothing with elastic for easier dressing.
- Switch from buttons to Velcro dots or magnetic closures.
- Like a belt with your outfit? Did you know that there are belts designed to clasp with one hand?
- Find clothing that won't easily get caught on a walker or wheelchair, which can become a dangerous tripping hazard.
- Select sturdy shoes with nonslip soles.

Don't let incontinence stop you

Another life-changing concern for men and women is incontinence, which is a very common—and often a very embarrassing—challenge for adults. Incontinence is such a tricky issue for many aging men and women that it can lead to self-isolation and can contribute to depression. First, incontinence is an important issue to address with your doctor, because there are many options for treating incontinence. Also, talk to therapists, caregivers or support groups to find comfortable, confident adaptations for living with incontinence.

There are hundreds of choices and designs and styles of adaptive gear, but start with these tips:

- Avoid too-tight clothing.
- Avoid zippers and buttons to ease undressing in the bathroom.
- Substitute Velcro in men's pants for buttons and zippers.
- Select clothing that washes well. Remember, even shoes can get wet. Look for easily washable shoes.
- Buy extra underwear and socks to cut down on the need to wash clothing so frequently.
- If you will be wearing an adaptive pad, garment or other gear, consider how your clothing will fit.

Helpful gear for confident living

There are thousands of adaptive items for confident living as we age and experience new limits or disabilities. Here are just a few ideas to start your discussion with family, friends and caregivers:

- Adult bibs, which allow for easy mealtime clean up, can become a fun part of your wardrobe. Does that seem impossible? You might be surprised at the fun and functional styles that many men and women enjoy wearing at mealtime. Got a favorite sports team? Get the bib! Got a favorite movie? Favorite celebrity? Fun message or famous quote? Get the gear!
- Bed pads, which can be washable or disposable, will limit your washing and cleaning chores.
- Wheelchair cushions with washable covers come in many shapes and sizes, including lumbar supports.
- Walker pouches, baskets and other brackets can carry frequently used items.
- Grabbers to reach out and pick up items come in a huge range of styles. When ordering, pay attention to the weight of the device. Can you lift and move it easily? What's on the grabbing end? Some have magnetic tips, perfect for picking up small metal items, like pins. Some have special rubber tips for picking up even the most delicate items. Consider getting more than one and keeping them handy around the house.
- Dressing sticks. These differ from grabbers and can become a very helpful tool for the independent person who has trouble dressing due to limited range of motion. Never heard of a dressing stick? Ask a therapist or watch online videos.
- Lap blankets are convenient for easily adapting to changing temperatures without having to fiddle with the thermostat.
- Non-slip socks and slippers can be lifesavers. Falling is one of the biggest threats to our health.
- Long-handled shoehorns are helpful for putting on shoes when you cannot bend at the waist.

- Zipper pulls give our fingers a larger surface to grab when using zippers.
- Button hooks sound like something used on shoes in Laura Ingalls Wilder novels, but they are cheap and handy for buttoning shirts.
- Wheelchair-friendly pants allow for easier assistance with dressing and bathroom use.
- Wheelchair gloves improve mobility.
- Need a new winter coat? Capes or ponchos are easier to manage than traditional jackets.

Please remember that this list is simply a starting point for you and your family. Occupational therapists are experts in a wide range of adaptive changes you can make to continue living independently. They can teach you how to dress, despite limited mobility, paralysis or neuropathy. They can also teach you how to use some of the gear you may wind up purchasing.

Finally, as we have already mentioned, discuss how often clothing will be laundered—and who will provide that service. Perhaps you are mobile enough to keep doing laundry. If so, discuss with your family and friends whether your washer and dryer should be moved to avoid falling hazards. Perhaps a relative or caregiver will be handling your laundry. Having enough clothes to make this a manageable, once-a-week task will help to keep those helpers from exhausting themselves on a daily basis.

This chapter is simply a starting point to make sure families are aware: You're never to old to dress for success.

16

Hidden Challenges and Helplines

Identifying easily overlooked issues before they become crises

This book is designed to empower individuals, families and friends to form caring communities that encourage healthy aging in place. Sometimes, however, we may stumble over hidden challenges that require new levels of care—or new kinds of expertise to successfully manage our daily lives.

In some cases, we need that outside help immediately!

This chapter identifies issues that may require new forms of assistance, perhaps involving medical specialists, treatments or training for yourself and your caregivers. Identifying these conditions may trigger a rethinking of our overall health care plan. We may need to start therapy, find additional equipment or perhaps make adaptations to our homes. This chapter is not an exhaustive list, of course, but it is a reminder to all of us that our goal of healthy aging in place requires honesty about easily overlooked issues that can turn into crises if we ignore them.

From tip to toes

Let's start with our extremities—our heads and feet.

Out of sight, out of mind, is not a healthy strategy for seniors who are more likely than the general population to develop treatable skin cancers or problems related to feet and toes. That's why an annual medical checkup often involves disrobing so the doctor can look over the trunk of your body and can examine your feet. This isn't an annoyance. It's good news, if an emerging issue is identified during your exam. That's because skin cancer and most foot problems are fairly easy to treat or manage—if these issues are caught early. Why would we ignore such issues? Because most of us rarely look at our backs, or the tops of our head where hair may have thinned, so we are likely to miss emerging spots that might be cancerous. In addition, as we age, a lack of flexibility may mean that we are unable to get a good look at our feet. So, if your annual exam includes a careful look at your skin and feet—thank your doctor for being thorough.

Don't worry too much about having these checks made. The risk of skin cancer rises as we age, but this form of cancer certainly is not inevitable. The vast majority of men and women never experience skin cancer. However, if newly emerging spots are identified—most can be treated or removed. You don't have to wait a year for a doctor to check. We now have more helpers watching over the skin of our head and shoulders. In many parts of the country, for example, hairdressers and barbers now are trained to ask about new growths they might spot as they regularly cut and style our hair. If a question is raised—go see a medical professional.

At the other end of our bodies—the range of potential foot problems fills entire podiatry textbooks. However, in simple terms, these issues fall into two general groups: First, *active* seniors can develop problems related to the aging tissues and circulation in our feet, making foot care an important part of our daily routine so we can keep using our feet for many years. Second, *inactive* seniors can develop problems by neglecting their feet. Plus, many chronic conditions, including diabetes and arthritis, can cause or complicate problems with our feet.

Among easy ways to reduce the likelihood of foot problems:

- Wear properly fitting, supportive shoes.
- Keep feet clean and moisturized.
- Clip nails.
- Watch and care for any sores.

- Watch and care for signs of fungus.
- Ask a professional about chronic pains, sores or fungi that aren't easily resolved.

Just because you can't see the top of your head, your back or your feet doesn't mean you can ignore them. If problems do develop, these conditions may require a visit to a specialist. Again: don't worry. If you're alert to problems and spot them early, most of these issues can be treated by your doctor.

Diabetes

We are including diabetes in this chapter because it is also frequently overlooked. Like skin cancer and foot problems, studies show that millions of Americans develop the condition known as prediabetes each year without realizing it. In fact, studies show that the majority of people with prediabetes are unaware of it until later and more serious problems arise. That is unfortunate, because steps can be taken when prediabetes is diagnosed—including changes in diet, weight loss and increased activity—that can prevent or delay diabetes from developing. If we don't realize we are prediabetic, we might not make such healthy choices early enough to avoid or delay diabetes.

The Centers for Disease Control (CDC) reports that nearly 1 in 10 Americans has diabetes, a condition that ranks among the leading causes of death in the U.S. The CDC warns: "Diabetes is a serious disease that can often be managed through physical activity, diet and the appropriate use of insulin and other medications to control blood sugar levels. People with diabetes are at increased risk of serious health complications including premature death, vision loss, heart disease, stroke, kidney failure, and amputation of toes, feet or legs."

Tests related to diabetes are a common part of a physical exam—one more reason to schedule these annual checkups even if you are feeling well.

Care to learn more? The American Diabetes Association has a web portal for seniors at www.diabetes.org/resources/seniors.

This nonprofit also maintains an informative helpline at 1-800-DIABETES (342-2383).

Substance abuse, mental health, suicide prevention

Substance abuse, alcoholism, addiction, mental health and suicide are complex issues. However, like the previous issues in this chapter, these problems often are ignored or overlooked in families until a crisis arises.

The good news is: Help is available.

All experts start with this advice: If someone is in a life-threatening situation, dial 911 now.

National Suicide Prevention Lifeline: By July 2022, the FCC is requiring all telephone service providers to route the phone number 988 to the National Suicide Prevention Lifeline. That national lifeline number has been 1-800-273-8255 (TALK)—a program maintained by the Substance Abuse and Mental Health Services Administration (SAMHSA), which is part of the U.S. Department of Health and Human Services. This National Suicide Prevention Lifeline connects callers with a network of local crisis centers that provides free and confidential emotional support to people in suicidal crisis or emotional distress 24 hours a day, 7 days a week.

Mental health and substance abuse national helpline: SAMHSA also maintains a second national helpline at 1-800-662-HELP (4357). This confidential information service is for individuals and family members facing mental health or substance abuse disorders. The helpline provides referrals "to local treatment facilities, support groups and community-based organizations. Callers can also order free publications and other information."

The complex challenges we are describing in this section often are interrelated and can be triggered by our own deep-seated psychological makeup, including trauma, as well as physical conditions, including genetic predisposition in some instances. While that may sound too complicated to identify, the fact is that many families watch evidence pile up over the years but ignore these signs with repeated excuses.

Among the most popular excuses:

- "Mom's lonely and enjoys a drink or two to take the edge off."
- "Sure, Dad has mentioned killing himself—but he would never do that. He's just down at the moment."
- "I don't know why Mom has started talking about something terrible that happened to her when she was a little girl. That was 50 years ago! I wish she'd just forget about it."
- "How often have we refilled his painkiller prescriptions? Shouldn't he be done with those meds? I guess his doctor knows what's good for him."
- "His friend gave him *what*?! I hope he's not regularly taking that. I guess he knows what he's doing."
- "Don't even try to phone him after 3 p.m. any day. By then, he's already started drinking. Just catch him in the morning."

All of these are serious warning signs that an intervention may be needed, perhaps starting with a visit to the doctor. One AARP report says that as many seniors are seen by medical professionals for alcohol-related crises as for heart attacks.

The majority of men and women over age 65 do not have problems with substance abuse, trauma or mental health. However, a significant but growing minority of seniors do wrestle with these issues. If you find yourself repeating common excuses like the ones listed above—instead, take compassionate action.

A special note on the lingering effects of trauma: Don't dismiss the warning signs just because a loved one seems too old to be suffering from traumatic injuries. Trauma can resurface as a powerful and crippling force even if the original crisis occurred many decades ago. In *Light Shines in the Darkness*, psychologist Lucille Sider writes about how the effects of childhood sexual abuse can resurface with a devastating impact even half a century or more after the original trauma. Counselors working with World War II veterans and Holocaust survivors have reported on the intense, lingering effects of trauma on men and women even as they reach their 90s. The same is true with military veterans, first responders and frontline medical personnel. Even professionals in the helping professions, such as teachers, social workers and pastors, may wind up suffering the effects of long-ago trauma in old age.

In at least some cases, our struggles with addiction, substance abuse, mental illness and trauma can contribute to suicidal thoughts. The most common myth families need to dispel is that someone who says they are contemplating suicide won't act on that impulse. A second common myth is that openly discussing suicide will contribute to the likelihood. Both of these myths lead to friends and family ignoring warning signs about suicide—either by dismissing a warning from our loved one or refusing to discuss the issue, once it is raised.

All of the national centers for suicide prevention urge honest conversation—and active interventions—to help anyone facing these often-overlooked challenges.

Getting a good night's sleep

According to the CDC, as many as 1 in 4 seniors do not get sufficient sleep, a condition that many families do not realize can have serious health consequences. Each person's need for sleep varies. Overall, however, the CDC says that most adults "need seven or more hours of sleep per night for the best health and well-being."

If you are experiencing chronic sleep problems, the CDC says "it is important to receive an evaluation by a health care provider or, if necessary, a provider specializing in sleep medicine." There are many ways professionals can help.

Among the most common problems related to sleep:

- Insomnia, the inability to fall asleep or to remain asleep for a healthy number of hours.
- Narcolepsy, excessive daytime sleepiness, weakness and sleeping.
- Sleep apnea, which can be characterized by snoring or gasping during sleep, or a lengthy pause in breathing—conditions that interrupt restful sleep and can result in excessive sleepiness throughout the day.

The CDC reports that sleep disorders are serious and research shows that they can increase the dangers of diabetes, cardiovascular disorders, obesity and depression.

Elder abuse

This hidden challenge is preventable, if we all work together to protect the most vulnerable in our communities.

Laws in a growing number of states now list caring professionals—including doctors and first responders as well as home health care providers—as "mandated reporters" of abuse or neglect they suspect is occurring. You may already have experienced an interaction with a professional asking such questions. For example, in many health care systems, a doctor or nurse may ask you, "Do you feel safe at home?" If you hear such a question, don't be defensive. Be honest. These are safeguards to help identify and stop abuse of vulnerable men and women.

The U.S. Department of Health and Human Services (HHS) begins its abuse-prevention presentations with the reminder we included earlier in this chapter: "Call 911 immediately if someone you know is in immediate, life-threatening danger." That's a warning well worth repeating.

What is elder abuse? The CDC and the HHS's Administration for Community Living (ACL) list seven forms of abuse:

- Physical Abuse—inflicting physical pain or injury on a senior, including slapping, bruising or restraining by physical or chemical means.
- Sexual Abuse—non-consensual sexual contact of any kind.
- Neglect—the failure by those responsible to provide food, shelter, health care or protection for a vulnerable elder.
- Exploitation or Financial Abuse—the illegal taking, misuse or concealment of funds, property or assets of a senior for someone else's benefit.
- Emotional Abuse—inflicting mental pain, anguish or distress on an elder person through verbal or nonverbal acts, including humiliating, intimidating or threatening.

- Abandonment—desertion of a vulnerable elder by anyone who has assumed the responsibility for care or custody of that person.
- Self-neglect—the failure of a person to perform essential, self-care tasks to the point that such failure threatens their own health or safety.

If the danger is not immediate, but you suspect that abuse has occurred or is occurring, HHS urges individuals, friends or family members: "Please tell someone. Relay your concerns to the local adult protective services, long-term care ombudsman, or the police."

Here's yet another option: Anywhere in the U.S., you can reach the Eldercare Locator at 1-800-677-1116. The Eldercare Locator is administered by The National Association of Area Agencies on Aging. Via the hotline, operators will refer you to a local agency that can help. The Eldercare Locator is open Monday through Friday, 9 a.m. to 8 p.m. Eastern time." You can also reach the Eldercare Locator at eldercare.acl.gov/Public/Index.aspx.

Dementia and Alzheimer's disease

Dementia is a broad range of brain disorders that limit the ability to think and remember to the point that our daily activities are compromised. Alzheimer's disease makes up more than half of all these cases in the United States, but dementia can also be caused by a long list of other disorders from vascular disease to HIV.

We are including a reminder in this particular chapter because Alzheimer's disease generally begins as a hidden disorder. The Alzheimer's Association, the largest nonprofit funder of research into the disease, warns families that the disorder may begin to develop as long as 20 years before symptoms are noticeable. Research continues, each year, on more accurate diagnostic tools for early screening. However, most individuals and families don't realize there is a problem until the disorder is well under way.

The most important advice from professionals is: If lapses in memory do become obvious, do not immediately assume a diagnosis of Alzheimer's disease. Consult a doctor. There may be other reasons one's memory is compromised, some of which are temporary and treatable.

Once again, there is a national helpline. The Alzheimer's Association maintains 1-800-272-3900, and describes the service this way: "Through this free service, specialists and master's-level clinicians offer confidential support and information to people living with the disease, caregivers, families and the public." However, all medical experts advise seeing your doctor as the first step in determining whether dementia is a chronic problem—and identifying what is causing this condition.

The CDC begins its introduction to families this way: "Alzheimer's disease is not a normal part of aging." More than 5 million Americans are living with Alzheimer's disease—but this disorder is not inevitable. To put this in perspective, experts point out that the majority of seniors living in the United States do not have—and will not develop—Alzheimer's disease. That's good news.

While there is no cure, there are risk factors that may contribute to the onset, including the aging process itself, diabetes, high blood pressure, smoking and a family history of dementia. The CDC urges everyone to be proactive about this disorder, advising families: "Researchers are studying whether education, diet and environment play a role in developing Alzheimer's disease. There is growing evidence that physical, mental and social activities may reduce the risk of Alzheimer's disease."

So, although this remains a scary, hidden disorder in many families, there is a lot you can do today:

- Get active and stay active.
- Manage cardiovascular risk factors, such as smoking, diabetes, hypertension and obesity.
- Learn new things each day.
- Stay connected with your family, friends and communities.

17

A Trip to the Doctor

Plan ahead to make the most of your health care team

One certainty as we age is that we will need to see health care professionals. Some of us rarely make medical appointments, while some of us need to see a whole list of specialists in an ongoing rotation. National averages suggest seniors see medical personnel about four times a year. All national health care organizations recommend that we should see a doctor at least once a year, even if we don't think we need to make such a visit.

There are many common reasons seniors avoid an annual checkup. The four frequently voiced excuses:

- We aren't noticing any symptoms, so we assume there's no point in having a checkup.
- We don't like or don't trust doctors.
- We don't have transportation.
- We can't afford a visit.

So, why should we see a doctor at least once a year? Here are some of the most common reasons listed by health care professionals:

- Many serious conditions can arise and grow without any symptoms appearing until these issues are acute and then are more difficult to treat. An annual checkup can catch a wide range of issues while they are more manageable.
- In particular, periodic scans and tests can catch cancers while they are relatively easy to treat.

- Regular contact with a doctor can help manage chronic problems like diabetes, high blood pressure and heart problems before debilitating effects arise.
- An annual checkup is a good time to go over our daily medications. We tend to accumulate medicines throughout a lifetime. Our doctor can help us weed out prescriptions that are no longer useful or that may conflict with other medicines.
- Sometimes medication levels need to be increased, changed or adjusted to prevent critical problems before they arise.
- An annual checkup provides baseline readings on our health, so doctors can more easily spot emerging problems over time.

Do you have to physically see a doctor?

An annual physical exam requires an office visit. But there are many instances where online connections are sufficient, especially if you have an ongoing relationship with a health care system. Throughout 2020, an enormous expansion of telemedicine rolled out nationwide. More doctors are also comfortable, now, interacting with patients and their designated representatives via secure emails or web-based exchanges. Beyond telemedicine, a wide array of medical devices—including smart devices we wear—now interact virtually with our health care providers.

However, remember: Many of these options depend on an already existing relationship with a health care system. That means an annual checkup is even more important. You will already be in your doctor's system, making virtual connections more practical.

Making the most of a trip to the doctor

Millions of older Americans make regular visits to a primary doctor as well as specialists for everything from hearing, vision and dental issues to chronic issues such as pain, diabetes, heart disease and cancer.

If you are planning a visit—either for yourself or an aging person in your care—start by asking simple questions:

- Why are you going to this appointment?
- What do you hope to accomplish?

Is this ...

- A post-surgery checkup?
- A periodic blood test or another form of screening?
- A visit to evaluate your health in light of a newly emerging symptom?
- A chance to discuss whether medications are working—or causing problems?
- An opportunity to renew soon-to-expire prescriptions?

Talk about the goals of the visit. Share questions and concerns and make a short list of the questions you hope to answer when you see the doctor and staff.

As needs of older adults increase, it may be necessary to identify a main health advocate. (Other chapters in this book describe the best way to organize your caregiving team and the most common legal documents that can make a person's choices clear even if that person becomes unable to clearly express preferences.) As a health advocate, your main role is to provide support and help coordinate care. You also are empowered to share the information gained at one appointment with any other doctors the older adult might see. A best practice is to stay organized. One way to do that is to incorporate the use of a folder or binder at all doctors' appointments.

Organizing your file for health care visits

Your folder or binder likely will include:

- Copy of the patient's ID.
- Copy of the patient's insurance card.
- Information about co-pays and costs to see a specialist.
- Phone numbers and contact information for all of the patient's doctors, including the purpose for seeing each one.
- A calendar of upcoming appointments so everyone is aware of ongoing treatments and visits.

- Phone numbers and contact information for the patient's preferred pharmacy.
- Approved health advocate information to make it clear that this person is empowered to speak with the doctor and staff— and can get information from test results.
- A list of all food and drug allergies.
- A complete list of all prescribed medications, over-the-counter medications, supplements and vitamins the patient is taking. You will want to include dosage, purpose, when the prescription was issued (and will expire) and side effects. A medication tracker worksheet could help to keep these up to date.
- Many pharmacies will also print off a list of all of a patient's prescriptions. You just have to make sure that you get such a list from every pharmacy the patient uses.
- A list of previously diagnosed conditions, surgeries, ongoing treatments and therapies—including when and why.
- Copies of any health-related legal documents, including advance directives, DNR, etc.
- Then, add an ongoing series of notes (or printed reports) to your file from visits, tests, etc.

Remember: Even your dentist, therapist or ophthalmologist will ask about much of the above information. So, carry this folder to all health care visits and be sure to update it at least once a year or when medications or health conditions change.

Tips on making the most of an appointment

You've already identified your companion, who serves mainly as a driver or friendly support for the visit—or may be a fully empowered health care advocate. As we age, it's best to have two people making these visits, if at all possible. Even if our memory is clear and our judgment is sound, health care visits often are fast and information is conveyed at a rapid pace. Terms are used that you may think you understand, until you are heading home and realize you should have asked about the words' exact meaning. A second person represents a second set of ears, another opportunity to have someone question a confusing term or clarify a complicated treatment. Sometimes flyers or informative papers are handed to the patient, and a companion represents a second set of eyes and hands to make sure everything is saved and carried home.

As you prepare for your visit, experts recommend:

- Make a list of questions for the doctor and staff.
- If there are changes to your address—or any of your contact information, including preferred phone number and email—write out that information in advance.
- Bring a log of problems or issues that may be occurring, including the timeline.
- Have a list of symptoms that may have started since last visit. Be able to verbalize when these symptoms are worse and what might relieve them.
- Be confident! Commit to asking for an explanation from the doctor of anything you don't understand. Don't feel embarrassed about asking more questions.
- As the appointment begins, be prepared to take notes. Consider recording the appointment so you and your caregivers can listen to it later—but be sure to ask for permission to make such a recording.
- Ask for the doctor, or staff, to provide written information about your condition, any treatment and follow up.
- Ask about side effects to newly prescribed medications and whether there are any instructions about when to take them. With a meal? Before bed?
- Ask about whether new medicines will interact with drugs or other pills or supplements you are taking. The staff may not be aware of everything you are taking. Bring out your current list from your file. See if your list matches what the staff has entered in their system.
- Ask how you will know when the new medication is working and how long should it take to start working.

- Discuss why the doctor is recommending a particular treatment—and if there are other treatment options.
- If an appointment with a new doctor is scheduled, ask for all the contact information you will need. Confirm all the details of the new appointment. Ask if your medical records are available to the new doctor.

The importance of regular medical screenings

Finally, here is a list of the most common kinds of screening recommended for all of us as we age:

- Cholesterol
- Blood pressure
- Diabetes
- Bone density
- Prostate
- Breast cancer
- Cervical cancer
- Colorectal cancer
- Mental health
- Sexual health
- Memory

This list can seem overwhelming, but it is an attempt to start the conversation with the primary care physician so that a comprehensive plan is made. This is one more reason that an annual checkup is helpful. Your doctor can help you to prioritize tests and screenings. Some of these may be recommended each year; others may not be necessary for many years. That checkup may turn out to be an annual source of relief and renewed confidence.

18

Directing Our Care

Advance directives, power of attorney, living wills and DNRs

As we grow older, we want to express our wishes for our final years—
and then trust that people will carry out these wishes even after we
are unable to do so. While some family members may feel anxious
about these discussions, or may even refuse to take part, the fact is
that a majority of aging men and women feel strongly about these
choices. They want reassurance that their wishes will be respected.

This chapter is not a substitute for legal advice. It's a helpful introduction to the basic tools families can use to carry out someone's
wishes. If you are interested in pursuing these options, consult an
attorney or explore some of the online links included at the end of
this chapter. Ask around your community. Some health care systems
and nonprofits provide free training.

One common headline for these programs is: "Have the
conversation!"

Or, as the Conversation Project, linked below, puts it: "Start your
conversation today."

Here's what you'll be talking about:

Advance directives

Too often we shy away from these discussions because they are
difficult to have, so some families wait until it is too late and the
person is no longer able to express their wishes.

Making decisions at the end of life can be difficult, scary and emotional, even with the proper documents in place. The types of advance directives people choose to make have names like DPOA, Living Will and DNR. Remember: Legally, you can change your mind and change the documents later. The key is to complete them in advance to prepare for a time when they are needed.

Brief Definitions:

- Durable Power of Attorney for Health Care (DPOA-HC) designates person(s) to make decisions for you when you are no longer able to make them. It must be signed and witnessed.

- POA (Power of Attorney) can be set up for non-health care reasons as well, such as to assist people with managing bills and other finances.

- Patient Advocate names the person(s) whom you designate to make your decisions. Other terms used includes medical decision maker, health care proxy or health care agent.

- Living Will is a document that provides guidance for future life-sustaining treatments. These are legal in some states but not all, but most DPOA-HC documents allow for including these wishes in the document.

- DNR (Do Not Resuscitate) form is usually signed by a patient and physician, then witnessed. A DNR order indicates that the person does not wish cardiopulmonary resuscitation (CPR) if their heart stops.

All states have durable powers of attorney for health care, with variations. Some states accept living wills as a separate document. In other states, those types of decisions are incorporated into the DPOA-HC. States also vary on how the document is to be activated. What is consistent across the board is that medical decision makers are intended to make decisions based on what they believe your wishes would be.

Because these documents vary across the 50 states, groups like AARP provide free materials for each state.

Durable power of attorney for health care (DPOA-HC)

What is important about this process?

- It gives you a decision maker in the hospital. Without one, sometimes hospitals have to determine who should make those decisions for you, or they go to court to have someone designated.
- If you don't have a document, and decisions need to be made, families may have to go to court to apply for guardianship, especially if there are disagreements among next of kin.
- Making a DPOA-HC better assures that the decisions you would want to make about your health care will be followed.
- These documents need to be made when a person is able to make their own decisions. Complete it sooner than later. If decision-making capacity diminishes there will be a point when the person no longer has the ability to complete such a form. If you wait for too long, the document could be challenged.
- Standard versions of these forms are readily available in your state and you can find them via your local hospital, the area Agency on Aging and AARP. You could use an elder-law attorney to create this document if you wish.

What should we consider?

- Pick someone who will make decisions based on your wishes. This may not be the oldest child, but the one who will be able to make the choices you would make.
- The decision-maker doesn't have to be a local person if someone who lives far away may better reflect your decisions or will have knowledge that you think would be helpful. Just one example: Your daughter in another part of the U.S. may be a nurse and may understand your wishes, making her the best person to designate, even though she does not live near you.
- Have at least two people if possible, listed in order. That way, if something happens to the first person, there is another

ready to take over. It is best to have the patient advocates in sequential order instead of requiring all decisions to be made conjointly. When someone is in the hospital with life or death decisions that need to be made, it is much easier for the hospital to contact one person rather than trying to get all parties in a room to make a decision.

- You may revoke or change your document. If possible, you should reread it and revise it periodically to make sure that your wishes are the same. One reason you might revise it is if the person you designated to make decisions is deceased or has developed dementia.

- Make copies and give them to family and those who are listed as patient advocates. Do not hide it in a drawer. Give a copy to your primary care provider and to your local hospital.

How to start the conversation

Having conversations with your family may be easier than you think. Every extended family is likely to have someone who is anxious and vocal about avoiding these subjects—but generally "the conversation" with your relatives winds up being more reassuring than you might expect.

Don't just write down your wishes, stick that paper in a drawer or in your favorite book and assume that you have completed your work. Having these conversations—especially with those who will likely be involved in making health care decisions—is just as important as expressing your wishes in writing. When facing end-of-life decisions, family members appreciate recalling previous conversations with you about these issues. This provides reassurance and greater certainty to those who are making difficult decisions.

What are good opportunities for starting a conversation?

- At or during a doctor's visit. As parents age, it is wise to seek permission to go to the doctor with them.

- When a relative is ill, explore with your loved one what they would choose in a similar situation.

- If someone expresses a concern or asks you about these issues, welcome the conversation.
- Check for local programs. Some health care systems and even a small but growing number of congregations offer counseling and support.

What topics should we include? Here are some questions that can prompt a helpful discussion:

- What gives you quality of life?
- What do you wish for comfort?
- How do you wish to be treated?
- How do you feel about life-support treatment?

This final question can get complicated because there are many types of treatment in this category, for example, tube feeding, blood transfusions, dialysis, IV antibiotics, etc. It may not be necessary to discuss each one separately, and it is virtually impossible to predict what issues decision makers will be facing in the future. It is better to have a general idea of how someone feels about life-support treatments.

In addition to the complex array of life-support treatments, this discussion takes time because a person's feeling about these treatments may vary depending on the situation. You may need to ask about specific cases:

- What if you are rushed to the emergency room?
- What if we know you are close to death?
- What if you are in a coma and doctors say you are unlikely to recover?
- What if doctors tell us there was brain damage?
- What if you develop dementia?

You can set up these documents to allow your advocate to make choices depending on the condition, situation and the levels of medical care involved. You also can express your wishes about being moved to a nursing home, hospice or hospital. You can make a point of empowering someone to advocate for better treatment.

Some of us don't want to get into that level of detail. Some of us prefer just to identify a trusted decision maker, then give them the documents so they can carry out that role.

Living wills

Living wills are legal in most states. Where they are not, most health providers will honor your wishes if they are written out and witnessed. Often, these wishes are incorporated into a DPOA. Living wills provide guidance for future life-sustaining treatments and can be quite detailed—or can give simple instructions.

Do Not Resuscitate (DNR)

This is a form that will address your outpatient wishes. The basic purpose of signing such a document is to let emergency medical providers (EMS) know that you do not want to be resuscitated if your heart and breathing should stop. Most states have DNR laws, although they differ in some states—and, a DNR order in one state may not transfer to a different state. These documents need to be completed with a physician who will need to sign the form. Some people will choose to complete this document at the same time as a durable power of attorney for health care, but they can also be completed at a later date.

Things to consider:

- For healthy younger people, a medical presumption would be that most people at this time in life would want to be resuscitated and, therefore, they do not put such documents into place. Physicians are unlikely to sign a DNR form in such a case.
- People often choose to make these documents near the end of life, when they are frail and are anticipating death.
- As we approach the end of life, the risks of CPR (cardiopulmonary resuscitation) increase, for example, causing broken ribs, or staying alive but without awareness or in a significantly reduced state.

- If you are no longer able to make this decision because you lack capacity (for example, you have dementia), your patient advocate may be able to make such a decision.
- DNR forms do no good unless they are accessible. Place them prominently where people will see them. Consider putting them on your refrigerator with other reminders you hang there, in your bathroom medicine cabinet or even on your front door. Give them to family members.
- Some states are now using a POLST form (Physician's Orders for Life-Sustaining Treatment), also called MOLST, MOST or POST, in addition to, or in place of, a DNR form. These are completed for individuals with a serious illness or advanced frailty near the end of life. The form serves as a medical order for specific medical treatments during a medical emergency and can include a do not resuscitate order. Often, they are initiated by the medical team. They work in conjunction with other advance directives.

What happens if you don't have these documents in place? You could find yourself in a situation that requires a probate court order to appoint a guardian, a state-appointed person who makes decisions about a person's body and health care. Many organizations advise avoiding guardianship if possible, as appointed guardians could be professionals, or total strangers. In some cases, guardians can greatly disrupt a person's life. In fact, some guardianships resulted in such negative experiences that the Michigan Attorney General's office launched a task force to examine and remodel the guardianship system. Ultimately, guardianship means a person loses the right to decide where they live, what treatment they receive, and sometimes even who they're allowed to see.

In summary, the best gift that you can give to those you love is to prepare for your care. Creating advance directives leaves a guide for your family and loved ones about the care you want for yourself. And, having as many conversations as possible ahead of time goes a long way in giving reassurance to family members and decision makers during crucial times that they are making the best decisions for you.

Additional resources

Visit these websites for additional information about directing care.

For more about the PREPARE program:
prepareforyourcare.org/welcome

For more about the Conversation Project:
theconversationproject.org/

For more about the Five Wishes approach: fivewishes.org/

For more about POLST and other related forms: polst.org/

Visit this website for free printable AARP advance directive
resources: www.aarp.org/caregiving/financial-legal/
free-printable-advance-directives/

19

Our Relationships

The people we meet define our lives

"We exist only in relation to our friends, family and life partners; to those we teach and mentor; to our co-workers, neighbors, strangers and even to forces we cannot fully conceive of, let alone define. In many ways, we are our relationships." Those are words of Derrick A. Bell, the first African American to serve as a tenured professor at Harvard Law School.

That says a lot: Existence is relationships. And these relationships can be even small ones.

This is a hopeful philosophy for aging people who seek the health benefits relationships can bring. With a lifetime of relationships large and small, as well as the skills of relationship building, this can be powerful medicine.

All it takes is some intentionality and imagination.

Finding the health benefits of being social

A healthy grandmother in her 80s had knee replacement surgery and followed doctor's orders while recuperating. Although she expected recovery to take a while, it was taking longer than expected. She realized she was isolated in her apartment. Several of her children, her most important relationships, visited often. But she missed her friends from playing bridge and going to church. She resumed those social relationships and her health immediately improved.

Families can become overwhelmed if they believe they are the only ones who can provide the social relationships elders need. As Bell argued, loose-tie relationships with neighbors and even strangers also provide the stuff of existence.

We can best help ourselves if we recognize the value in all kinds of relationships, including those that are casual, new, temporary and nontraditional.

New, nontraditional relationships

A newspaper editor born in 1929, the same Depression year as the bridge-playing grandmother, is one of the mentors Bell mentioned. The editor worked in newsrooms for 58 years, long past retirement age. He downsized, took a pay cut, didn't mind. He liked the atmosphere and he loved to mentor young people.

The central relationship in his life was his college sweetheart. Their marriage was in its seventh decade. But in their 80s, Alzheimer's muted the last few years of the relationship. Although she no longer knew who he was, the editor continued to visit his wife several times a week.

There was no dissonance when, with a twinkle behind his thick glasses, he talked about his new "girlfriend." Ever the teacher, he helped his friend learn English. She taught him a few words of Vietnamese and introduced him to new cuisine. Their relationship did not supersede or negate the one he had with his wife, to whom he remained faithful. There is room in us for relationships of many kinds, even ones for which there is no handy name.

Who's your support squad?

This book describes the dangers of social isolation or seclusion. Once you accept the idea that your relationships need not all be the traditional go-to people, such as family, you can search further. Your inventory of possible relationships can include old friends and new ones, close ones and second- or third-degree connections. The possibilities will surprise you.

Mine your networks, choosing a few people from each area. You can start with:

- Family
- People you see every day
- Neighbors
- People with shared interests or hobbies
- The people in your address book or mailing lists
- People who call you
- People at your place of worship
- Co-workers and old schoolmates from long ago

The networks keep us healthy and active. Building them requires intentionality. Once we have a list of prospects, we need to start reaching out. We do not need an elaborate plan, but we need to cultivate them.

The *San Antonio Express-News* published an article by Richard A. Marini about how pandemic stay-at-home orders sparked a surge in phone calls. Stuck inside, people reached out.

One 84-year-old grandmother described a family-centric plan. With five grandchildren and seven great-grandchildren, she simply but deliberately calls one person a day. She focuses on the younger ones, whose lives she finds most interesting. She deliberately built a network that is age-diverse, a good strategy.

Marini also wrote about Ray Fuller, a retired web designer. Fuller began going through the contacts in his phone and calling people he hadn't spoken to in a while.

Marini wrote that Fuller talked to former work colleagues, the widow of a friend he didn't know had died and a friend living in an apartment by himself.

Fuller told Marini, "I tried calling another friend I've known since we were 10 years old. But when he didn't answer, I texted his wife. When we finally connected, we talked for, like, an hour and a half."

Fuller said he was using a lesson he learned when he had a cancer scare. "A lot of people wouldn't call me because they thought it was a private thing," he said. "But whenever a friend would call, it made me feel pretty good. So that's why I do it now."

Fuller is saying that we are not taking advantage of people when we reach out to people to help us feel connected. The contact can be a lifeline for someone else.

A range of perspectives makes better teams

In Kansas, National Teacher of the Year Tabatha Rosproy teaches 16 preschoolers in a classroom inside a retirement community. Rosproy and her intergenerational program were profiled by national reporter Kalyn Belsha on the education news website Chalkbeat.org.

Rosproy said that when the generations meet, students get read to in the lap of their grandparents-for-a-day and the elders go to the playground with the children, jump in puddles and play Bingo with them.

Stay-at-home orders stopped that. So, Rosproy has the students mail letters and pictures. She has tried window visits and made a video so the children could send their messages to their much-older friends.

Fuller and Rosproy have been creative in using resources that are close at hand. They also created connections that mean something to both parties. They crossed barriers of age, distance and even the distance that can grow during a long absence. They bridged them all.

Think of your network as a coaching staff. In baseball, the manager leads the team, but also has coaches for pitching, batting and fielding. As you build your network, have you covered all your bases? Is there someone you can engage with on faith? Finances? Health? Are there people to talk with about your various interests? It takes a well-rounded coaching staff to do all this.

It might also help to have a friend outside the family who can be a listening ear for family issues.

Pets can be part of healthy networks, too

Relationships need not always be the human kind.

A 2019 research article about older people and pets found these relationships can be very rewarding. However, the authors cautioned about potential challenges.

The researchers noted that older Baby Boomers face diminishing social networks, smaller and more dispersed families. They reported that pets give people companionship, structure, safety and social interactions with other pet owners.

However, pets must be chosen with consideration for the owner's fiscal and physical ability to care for their companions.

To one degree or another, pets can provide some of the relationships that keep us healthy.

"We help each other"

Remember the grandmother with the new knee? She became a great-grandmother, traded her car keys for a walker and moved from her apartment into assisted living. When the COVID-19 pandemic hit, she was 91 and isolated again. Her children and grandchildren were not allowed in; she could not leave. They tried to talk through the closed glass door, but masks muffle voices.

During the pandemic, the federal Health Resources and Services Administration tied weak social relationships to a 29% increase in the risk of coronary heart disease and a 32% rise in the risk of strokes.

AARP advised that social isolation could protect you from the coronavirus—but that "a recent scientific report elevates social isolation and loneliness to the level of health problems …"

Many older people are frustrated. It is risky to be exposed to the disease and risky to be isolated because of it.

In weekly Zoom reunions on her iPad, the great-grandmother told her children about painting and playing Scrabble with new friends and plotting to bend social-distancing rules that prevented more than two people from being together. "It's better to ask for forgiveness than to ask for permission," she told her children.

Sometimes, she was the one who ended the Zoom reunions. She regularly walks the grounds with Bill, a friend from high school who also lived there and who has lost most of his vision. "We help each other," she said.

Her friends, the new ones and the long-standing ones, did not replace her family. But they provided some of the vital relationships she needed to beat isolation, to recover from things like knee surgery—and to enjoy health and happiness.

20

Enjoying Life

Having fun is healthy!

Pursuing our hobbies and interests is good for our health!

Even the most well-organized among us can forget to take some time out of the day to enjoy life after completing our lists of routine self-care and maintenance. Graceful aging doesn't mean giving up the things we enjoy—we're actually more prepared than ever before to accomplish our personal goals and have fun with our favorite activities.

To make sure you are able to safely enjoy your favorite crafts, hobbies, physical activities and entertainment, plan ahead for any accommodations or safety guidelines you'll need to follow. It can also help to write them down in a journal or daily log. This preparation will help you incorporate having fun into your daily routine.

Getting older doesn't mean we have to give up our favorite pursuits. If anything, we can draw on a rich lifetime of experience to enhance them. The first step to enjoying—or getting reacquainted—with our personal interests is to determine any age-appropriate adjustments we need to make. That can include making any necessary accessibility modifications ahead of time, including online setup, and checking for the availability of age-appropriate resources.

For stories of real men and women who kept going with their favorite pursuits on a daily basis, see Chapter 4: Our Gifts. In particular, our favorite physical disciplines—from dance and yoga to sports—can ensure exceptional flexibility and longevity. Sometimes, adaptations lead to unexpected pleasures. Chapter 4 includes the story of Anna Mary Robertson Moses who had to give up her hobby of embroidery, because she could no longer manipulate her needles. That didn't stop her for a moment. Her passion was art. Instead of embroidering pictures, "Grandma" Moses began to paint—and the rest … is history.

For ideas of service as a vocation in our later years, see Chapter 5: Our Service. In that chapter, you will read: "Community service is, at its core, about giving of ourselves to address a pressing need we share with our neighbors. It is compassion in action. Through compassion, we connect at the deepest level to one another and can create meaningful change."

Life after 65 often gives us a wide range of opportunities we may never have experienced earlier in life. So, let's have some fun!

Media and accessibility resources

Love to read or enjoy favorite films and TV shows? Even if your hearing, eyesight or dexterity aren't what they used to be, many government programs and nonprofits—especially public libraries—offer adaptive resources for continuing to enjoy newspapers, magazines, books, TV and movies. These resources include captioned media, audio recordings and alternate formatting, like large print or dialogue-emphasized volume in audio and video streaming. Consider visiting your local library online or in person to learn about their resources. Ask a friend or family member to help you get connected, or ask your local librarian to show you around.

Libraries have vastly expanded their multimedia resources. For example, if you enjoy a particular kind of movie or TV series—perhaps from a particular era or genre or language or nationality—most public libraries now offer a wide range of choices. Talk to a librarian about how you'd like to receive such media.

Look carefully at the options built into the devices in your home—or ask for help from a tech-savvy friend or relative. One common adaptive option comes as a component included in many new TV sets: You can access the TV's audio settings and choose an option to have dialogue enhanced in the overall volume. Are you having trouble distinguishing some words in TV dialogue, when it's mixed with the other background sounds and music? Adjusting this setting can make a world of difference in clearly hearing your favorite TV characters.

Do you enjoy taking classes? There are many free, or low cost, in-person classes at nonprofit centers, congregations and community colleges. Not sure what course to take? Consider learning a skill like creative writing or event planning—or learning how to play a new game, like a board or card game. Learning a skill pays multiple dividends by allowing you to move from basic training to joining a local group of other like-minded people to enjoy your new abilities. If you learn to play a card game, you can join a card club. If you learn needlework or woodwork, you can join a crafting group.

Are you unable to attend in person? Many libraries now offer free access to online classes. A librarian can help you figure out the best way to receive them and actively participate.

Among the most common excuses for avoiding these enjoyable opportunities: "Oh, I just can't do that anymore." Most seniors are startled to learn about the full array of adaptive devices that can help them to keep enjoying their favorite pursuits. For example, if you enjoy listening to audio books, you can access them now on the smartphone you hold in your hand. So, you may not need any additional equipment to keep enjoying the authors and genres you love. Just ask around about how to find free audiobooks online. If you are unable to manipulate a smartphone, or don't own one—ask for help. There are media solutions for all forms of disability.

Is your favorite reading the daily news? Many public radio stations and universities broadcast a radio reading service for daily news, books and other media for people who may have trouble accessing or reading printed text. Many of these services also stream online and provide affordable or free radio service across the internet. Does finding these services seem daunting to you? The next time a media savvy friend or relative pays a visit, make this your activity for the afternoon. Your friend most likely will enjoy sampling various options with you and talking about which ones you might like to receive on a regular basis. Also note: Many of these services also archive previous broadcasts, allowing for hours for enjoyable listening even after the daily broadcast is over.

Age-appropriate exercise programs

Sports and exercise are great mood boosters and keep you healthy. Research shows exercise is also important for reducing cognitive decline that can occur with age. Whether you enjoy going for a walk or want to play in an age-appropriate soccer league, there are free or affordable resources and programs available to you. Consider joining a local walking group, an exercise class or sports league. You can find out about these groups and classes through social media, community gathering places near your home, your place of worship or even your local senior center. Many municipalities also offer adult fitness classes through their community education programs.

Visit this website to use AARP's localized activity finder: local.aarp.org

It's fun to try new activities. Consider crafts, sports and hobbies that take you outside, provide a little bit of exercise and let you meet new people. These might include bird watching, exploring your local arboretum or park, or participating in outdoor activities sponsored by your city or county.

Online fun

Going online is a great way to stay in touch with friends and family during your day-to-day activities. See Chapter 7: Going Online, for more tips.

This can include spending time on video chat while you do chores—from gardening outdoors to cooking in the kitchen. You can play virtual board games together, like Scrabble or Yahtzee. It's true that many of the first offerings you'll find online may cost money—but keep looking. There are free options for both video chatting and board games. Ask your friends and family to help you get set up.

Many families enjoy sharing a meal even if they're no longer living in the same home. Consider setting up a video chat date to cook or eat together. You can even have a virtual movie night by synchronizing your favorite streaming service to make sure you're watching the same movie at the exact same time. Check out services like www. netflixparty.com to get started.

The sky's the limit—literally!

Read Chapter 4 to learn about a man who finally had the time to prepare for flying after he retired—and earned his pilot's license at age 80.

We may be limited by our health and household budgets—but we aren't limited by our past experiences. As you envision your future, dare to choose activities that will make you happy. You deserve some joy!

To help you brainstorm, here are some of the most popular activities among seniors nationwide:

- Volunteering tops the list! See Chapter 5.
- Walking regularly is a close second—and consider building up your endurance for more ambitious hiking in parks and wilderness areas.
- Caring for animals ranks very high, as well. Even if you don't want to have your own pet, consider becoming a dog trainer, dog walker or regularly volunteering to foster or provide vacation care for other people's pets.
- Training in yoga or another physical-spiritual discipline such as Tai Chi.
- Learning a new sport—there are dozens of choices, from pickleball and bowling to croquet and table tennis.
- Learning video games.
- Gardening.
- Singing—either on your own or join a local choir.
- Writing your own songs or poetry or stories.
- Practicing a musical instrument.

- Joining a local theater group.
- Volunteering at a local public radio or TV station.
- Joining a book club.
- Dancing.
- Researching genealogy—See Chapter 21: Our Story, Our Legacy.
- Building models.
- Painting.
- Birding.
- Camping.
- Geocaching.
- Practicing photography and related skills—scrapbooking, picture framing, self-publishing.
- Learning about astronomy and star-gazing.
- Writing.
- Solving puzzles—from crosswords to jigsaw puzzles.
- Restoring historic furniture or even an entire house.
- Training as a docent at a local museum or historic site.
- Keep learning—take an affordable class at a community college or through your library or congregation.
- Teaching—lead a class focused on your own expertise.
- Traveling—finally you may find yourself free of scheduling restraints, so enjoy that new freedom.
- Learning a new craft—make pottery, stained glass windows or bonsai plantings; or think about hooking rugs, arranging flowers or scrapbooking.
- Learning a new language—yes, it is possible well after 65 and, in fact, this is one of the most popular activities among seniors.
- Starting your own coffee group and brainstorming even more ideas!

21

Our Story, Our Legacy

What do you hope people will remember about you?

What do you hope people will remember about you when you're gone?

Is it your cooking? What about your sense of humor? Perhaps you're most proud of your civic or military service.

We each spend a lifetime curating the story of "me." We bring signature dishes to every family gathering; we write heartfelt or humorous notes and greeting cards; we display collections from our birthplace, our travels; we teach young people our favorite games (as if they ever had hope of besting us); we point to this photo or that vase and tell a story for the tenth or hundredth time.

But as we age, we must teach others to be the keepers of our stories. The best way to do that is to leave behind tangible reminders of the most important parts of our lives. This is the literal definition of legacy: something handed down.

Reflect for a moment on how you'd like to be remembered, then consider: What can you leave behind to remind family, friends and even future generations of you? In this chapter, you will find practical ideas for preserving our stories.

You may be surprised to find museums, nonprofits or other organizations interested in your life experiences. You may also be surprised by simply asking loved ones now what stories they would like to hear again, what memories you haven't yet shared, or what skills they wish you would teach. Let the steps presented here open conversations and lead to requests for help. The most meaningful way you can pass down your story is to enlist others in preserving it.

Where is everything?

If you've ever moved from one home to another, then you know how challenging it can be to find and reorganize scattered, important documents and keepsakes. Now imagine a family member or even a stranger trying to accomplish that task for you. Do you think they would find everything? Would they understand the significance of certain items? Is there any room for misinterpreting your wishes?

The reality is that huge amounts of "important papers" get heaved into trash bins—even beloved family photo albums and priceless keepsakes like medals or great-grandma's recipe cards—when a sudden illness, move or death requires people to empty out a home in a hurry. You know that shoebox in your closet where you safely tucked away a few precious papers, letters and photos from an ancestor? In a speedy cleanup, that box will look like all the other old shoeboxes that are quickly tossed into a giant dumpster. Yes, your mom's beloved Bible is right there on the bookshelf, but a clean-up crew may shovel it—and all the little notes and gems inside her Bible—into a big box of dusty old books headed to a Salvation Army drop-off center.

There are even Facebook groups trying to unite families with long lost photos that have found their way through secondhand shops. That's why this first section is designed to help you to be proactive in organizing and preserving special family papers and other items.

The information here is presented in three tiers:

- Documents you must keep for legal or financial reasons,
- Documents you may wish to preserve for the future,
- And items you can consider passing down now.

Things to keep

Personal finance expert Dave Ramsey has a comprehensive guide to the paperwork you should keep, and for how long. www.daveramsey. com/blog/organizing-your-important-documents

He recommends gathering absolutely everything you have and organizing it into five keep piles based on the length of time you need to retain them:

1. Trash now
2. 1-3 months
3. 1 year
4. 7 years
5. Indefinitely.

If you follow this system, your "Keep Indefinitely" pile will contain most of the documents that are important for final affairs.

If you want to go one step further to aid family or friends in the event of your death, many insurance companies have guides to preserving the information required to settle your estate. Look around the websites of such long-standing companies, such as Allstate or State Farm, and you will find free, downloadable checklists for gathering essential contact information, account numbers, access to digital accounts and significant dates in one place.

Anything you gather in this category should be stored in a safe place, away from moisture. If possible, also consider a locked, fireproof safe—or a safety deposit box at a bank. If you do share a backup copy with a trusted relative, make sure to keep a list of where any copies have gone, what dates they were shared—and where they can be found.

Another option to consider is an online organizing service. Everplans, LifeSite, Yourefolio and Afternote are all online platforms which allow you to upload, store, and easily share access to wills, insurance policies, directives, funeral wishes and medical documents. Even if you don't choose to use their service, they also provide free guides and checklists about what to keep and how to store it.

Things to preserve

After you preserve the essential documents, you may realize how much more you have that is meaningful in your life. What about photographs, newspaper clippings, telegrams, letters, school or service records, even journals? The Society of California Archivists has compiled specific storage tips for these precious items. Look for resources at their website: calarchivists.org.

As we will explore a little later in the chapter, these items may be of interest to museums, archives, or historical societies, not to mention your loved ones. Take steps to keep them safe.

At the very least, if you want to avoid having family photos discarded you should label them. Consider a note on the back identifying the people in the picture, the occasion and the date if possible. Your family is much more likely to hold onto them if they understand the significance of the images. Of course, there are digital services to assist in this work too. Savefamilyphotos.com has tips on restoration and digitization. Again, this is a step you don't have to take alone. You don't even have to tackle it all at once. The next time you pull out an album to share, take an extra minute to make notes on the pictures.

Things to pass down

For some people, the idea of having their possessions distributed after death is unpleasant—especially when it seems they will be reduced to their material value. Consider the unique opportunity you have to gift items with a story now, rather than simply naming them in your will. By writing down the family history of an object—the special occasions when it was bought, gifted or used—you give your loved one something to cherish. This can be a great way to strengthen your relationship. Plus, you get to hear their thank-yous about any new memories created as you pass down the keepsake!

When you have a particular recipient in mind, write them a personal letter about the item. You can gift it on a special occasion or simply their next visit. Otherwise consider writing general notes for items you are already planning to store until later. The care you take now ensures that care will be taken to place the item in its next loving home.

Genealogy

All of us wish we knew more about our families. Sometimes, sharing our stories with each other is enough. However, millions of men and women around the world like to dig even deeper.

Genealogy is the study of families, family history and the tracing of their lineages. More than just "who's who" in your family tree, it can tell you a lot about your ancestors' lives, occupations and connections to historically significant people or events. In China, the recording of genealogies called Jia Pu started in the mid-1600s and complete records can span 10 volumes. Māori people learn to recite their whakapapa, an oral genealogy that links them as an individual to the land and their tribe. In 2019, Ghana started a "Year of Return" initiative to encourage Black Americans to repatriate to Africa, acknowledging that many may not be able to trace their family history through slavery back to their country of origin.

Genealogies have always held significance, across cultures and continents. No matter the family, undertaking this kind of research is a precious gift of time and persistence. If you want to get started, the National Archives has a comprehensive list of online sources. There are guides on how to do genealogical research, helpful sites and searchable document databases. Other free or low-cost resources include local libraries and historical societies, state archives, and FamilySearch.org, a site provided by The Church of Jesus Christ of Latter-day Saints. No matter where you start, keep these general tips in mind:

- Work from known information to unknown. Write down names, relationships, dates and places that you are sure are accurate, and use those to verify any new information you find.
- Start with sources in your own home and work outward.
- Decide what you want to research. Pick some key questions you want to answer about your family history and pursue those. This will keep you focused and enable you to filter out a lot of extraneous information.

- Print it out—or write it down. However you choose to create your saved record, make sure to save notes on your research along the way. Keep a record of key facts and which reference documents support each piece of information.

- Be sure you know how you found your way through a particular search. If not, you may be disappointed later that you simply cannot find the circuitous path you followed, especially in online research.

- Be critical. You must interpret all of the information you find to decide whether it is credible or correct. The increased interest in creating family trees on public sources like Ancestry, mean a lot of people are entering information who have different standards for verifying information. Even primary records are prone to errors like misspellings, incorrect dates, or poor translations.

Perhaps you've undertaken some family research and hit a wall, or perhaps the mere idea of starting is overwhelming. In that case, you may consider hiring a professional. Professional genealogists are already well versed in the best research practices, which sources are reliable, and how to be efficient in their work. You can locate professionals through the two major consumer genealogy sites: Ancestry and FamilySearch, or through the credentialing organizations listed by FamilySearch. Both websites also offer helpful tips about hiring professionals. You might especially consider a professional if your family originated in another country where records may be in a foreign language. They simply have wider ranging, established professional networks to accomplish more difficult research tasks.

It has become increasingly popular to start or supplement family history research with genetic information. One note of caution: Use of the most popular DNA testing (and public family tree research) services can expose deeply personal information online. You ought to be prepared to find connections you weren't anticipating. The interpretation of genetic ancestry information is also continuously evolving. Not all tests are equally reliable. The National Library of Medicine, a branch of the National Institute of Health, has a group of resources to aid in understanding test results at ghr.nlm.nih.gov/primer/dtcgenetictesting/ancestrytesting.

You don't need to trace your family all the way back to the 1600s or your genetic origins in order for your search to be worthwhile. Even delving back just one or two generations can reveal details, like former addresses or occupations or military service that help you see your history in a new light.

Your story may interest others

As you've organized your own papers and explored your family history, you may wonder if some of what you uncover has significance beyond your family and loved ones. Are you a candidate for an archive? A surprising number of people have personal papers that a regional archive may want to save. You don't have to be "famous" for an archive to want your materials. Here are just a few of the questions an archivist might ask:

- Do you have records of a social organization, fraternity, club, congregation or union that might interest researchers? Perhaps you or an ancestor served as the secretary for a club for recent immigrants from some part of the world?
- Got letters sent home to you by someone serving in the armed forces?
- Got a detailed diary of your work in a particular profession?
- Did you wind up with boxes of the founding papers from a community nonprofit you ran?

Almost every town is interested in documents related to its civic and cultural life. It's worth asking at a local library or historical society about their archives. An archivist can ask questions and help you determine if something you've saved would be of interest to other people in a public collection.

If you've lived through a larger moment in history, you should look further for regional or national archives. Many universities have special research interests for which they maintain archives. A simple internet search of the name of the university plus "archive" should help lead you to the categories in which they specialize.

There is significant interest at all levels in the histories of marginalized people or groups. In these cases especially, archives are seeking oral histories. According to the Oral History Association (OHA): "Oral history is a field of study and a method of gathering, preserving and interpreting the voices and memories of people, communities, and participants in past events. Oral history is both the oldest type of historical inquiry, predating the written word, and one of the most modern, initiated with tape recorders in the 1940s and now using 21st-century digital technologies." Similar to genealogical research, your oral history is worth recording even if it never goes further than your own family. The OHA website has free webinars and a list of links to oral history programs around the world to help you get started. The UCLA library has also compiled a guide for family members taking oral histories from their own relatives. Taking an oral history requires in-depth preparation on the part of the interviewer, designed to get as much engagement from the interview subject as possible.

We hope this chapter is inspiring you to organize and preserve a fuller picture of your life as a rich legacy to family, friends and the community. Any way in which you can gift your story is significant.

Overwhelmed with all of these suggestions? Start small. Set a goal of doing one thing each day. Label some pictures, annotate a favorite recipe, write a dedication in a favorite book, or pass on a small item.

You'll be smiling when you see all the smiles you inspire in others.

Additional resources

For more about preparing to take oral history, visit the following websites:

www.oralhistory.org/about/do-oral-history/

www.library.ucla.edu/destination/center-oral-history-research/ resources/conducting-oral-histories-family-members

www.oralhistory.org/about/principles-and-practices-revised-2009/

www.oralhistory.org/web-guides-to-doing-oral-history/

22

What Is Hospice Care?

Finding comfort and peace at the end of life

Hospice.

To some, that's a dirty word. Many families don't even want to utter the word.

But to millions of families who understand hospice—and have used its full array of services—"hospice" implies comfort, peace and love.

Hospice professionals understand both experiences. They understand that, when they pay a visit, some relatives or friends may not warmly accept them. They understand that, first and foremost, their mission is to meet every individual where they are emotionally, psychologically and spiritually.

Family conversations about hospice care can produce a great deal of anxiety—even outright terror. Families are coming to terms with the reality of death.

Rabbi Joseph Krakoff, director of Spiritual Care at Michigan-based Jewish Hospice and Chaplaincy Network, recalls a particularly challenging visit:

> I was visiting an 80-year-old man who had been diagnosed with stage 4 cancer. His three adult children had made an executive decision not to tell their father that he was dying. They also were adamant about not informing him that he was receiving hospice care. On my first visit,

the three siblings greeted me in the foyer of the man's home to firmly instruct me not to tell their father that he was on hospice. While I accommodated their request—I did so reluctantly. It was on my fourth visit to his home though, that without warning, he asked his children to leave because he wanted to speak to me alone.

The man beckoned me to sit down next to him on the chair by his bed and went on to speak the following words unequivocally: "Rabbi, my family thinks that I don't know what is going on. But I do! I recognize that I am dying and know I am on hospice. I have lived a very good life and realize my time here is short. I can get my head around that. What I struggle with the most though is that I really want to talk about my hospice care and the fact that I am dying, but my children won't allow it. Please help me help them to talk about it. I need to get my affairs in order. Even more, I want the chance to say goodbye to each family member individually and to express my gratitude and love for them. Rabbi, I beg you to help me with my kids."

Although the dialogue is slightly different, this situation is not an uncommon occurrence. What I find with some regularity is that people who are dying absolutely want to talk about it. And to them, hospice is not a bad word. Rather, it is a word that recognizes with honesty that they have entered the final chapter of their lives and they have chosen a compassionate, thoughtful and patient-centered approach to their care. And making this choice is sometimes the only control that remains when it seems that all other decisions they could make about their lives have ceased to exist.

Krakoff speaks and writes nationally about end-of-life issues. He always emphasizes that hospice has deep roots in our shared Jewish-Christian-Muslim heritage, reaching all the way back to the time of Jacob. Here is how Rabbi Krakoff tells the story:

> To truly understand the life-affirming values associated with hospice care, think about the very first occurrence of human illness mentioned in the Bible. In Genesis 48:1 we learn that the patriarch Jacob nears the end of his life. His son Joseph is immediately informed that his father is terminally ill. The Jewish oral tradition, trying to interpret Jacob's response to his own mortality, is preserved in Jewish tradition in what is known as the Midrash of Pirkei D'Rabbi Eliezer, Chapter 52:
>
> "From the days of Creation, a person had never become ill. Rather, if he was walking on the road or in the marketplace he would sneeze and his soul would depart through his nostrils, until our forefather Jacob asked the Almighty for compassion. Jacob prayed: 'Master of the Universe, do not take my soul from me until I instruct my children and grandchildren.'
>
> In this rabbinic story, we come to understand that Jacob asked God not to spare his life—but to both give him the opportunity to get his affairs in order and to bid farewell to his loved ones. This, in short, is a huge benefit that hospice care can provide: We give family members and friends the opportunity to engage in a meaningful goodbye.

The word hospice originated in medieval times, a derivative of the Latin *hospes*, meaning host or guest. It's the same Latin root that developed into the English terms we use today for hospitality, hotel, hostel and hospital. The history of hospitals stretches back more than a thousand years.

Hospice as a concept we recognize today appears initially in the mid-1800s to describe caring for dying patients and is based on the model created by Mrs. Jeanne Garnier, the founder of the Dames de Calaire in Lyon, France. It is said that the Irish Sisters of Charity adopted it when they created Our Lady's Hospice in Dublin, Ireland, in 1879 and then again when they opened St. Joseph's Hospice in Hackney, London, England, in 1905.

It wasn't until 1974 though that the first hospice was established in the United States.

Now, hospice is available through Medicare to critically ill patients who are declining and expected to die within six months. They agree to forgo any kind of aggressive medical intervention, including curative treatment. The vast majority of hospice is covered by Medicare, though some is paid for by private insurance, Medicaid and the Department of Veterans Affairs.

Agencies receive nearly $16 billion a year in federal Medicare dollars to employ nurses, social workers and aides to care for patients wherever they live. To get paid a daily fee by Medicare, hospice agencies must develop a care plan for each patient and be on call 24 hours a day, 7 days a week.

No, you're not 'giving up'

One of the biggest misnomers about hospice care is that accepting a referral to hospice means that the individual is "throwing in the towel" and giving up on life. For this reason, it is not unusual that people may be discouraged by family members to invoke their hospice benefit. But when the medical team determines that there is nothing else they can do and the terminally ill person is psychologically ready, then hospice can be the best choice, for it is particularly effective for reducing physical pain, maximizing emotional well-being and enhancing spiritual peace.

It is important to be clear that entering hospice is never a sign of weakness and it should not be a source of guilt. It is not giving up. Instead, it is about deciding to focus on the quality of life for whatever time is left.

We often see that someone on hospice actually begins to feel better or improves due to the extra layer of care provided by the hospice team composed of nurses, aides, social workers, clergy and volunteers. Many individuals on hospice actually live much longer than six months and some even graduate from hospice if their health stabilizes.

In choosing hospice, the individual has made the decision, in the event of a crisis, not to go to the hospital and not to call 911. Rather, all phone calls are made to the hospice organization no matter the time of day or night. And if, for whatever reason, a person changes their mind, they always maintain the authority to revoke their hospice benefit and revert to calling 911, going to the hospital and pursuing treatment.

It is no secret that the cultural situation in the United States often results in us consciously avoiding discussing end of life realities. Hospice clergy and other staff are trained to discuss this topic and sometimes pose very hard questions. In providing spiritual care to a patient considering hospice care and/or confronting the end of life, a hospice professional may ask questions such as:

- If you were not able to do the activities you enjoy, are there any medical treatments that would be too much?
- If you had to choose between living longer or having a higher quality of life, which would you pick?
- How important is it for you to live as long as possible, even if it means that you would experience pain and suffering?
- What fears do you have about dying?
- Do you want to die at home?

Dr. Ira Byock in his essay "Dying Shouldn't Be So Brutal" explains that "people who are approaching end of life deserve the security of confident, skillful attention to their physical comfort, emotional well-being and sense of personal dignity ... Most people want to drift gently from life, optimally at home, surrounded by the people they love."

Over the past half century, hospice care has spread across the United States. Now, there are more than 5,000 hospices in the U.S. serving more than a million people.

They share core values, usually listed on each hospice website. As one example, the Jewish Hospice and Chaplaincy Network in West Bloomfield, Michigan, describes its mission this way:

Our work is crafted around the belief that terminally ill patients want assurance of five things:

- To be free of pain
- To be respected and not treated as a burden
- To feel loved
- To not be alone
- To be remembered.

While we know there always will be some resistance to discussing hospice, the truth is that hospice care wholly focused on comfort and peace can be a true gift. Hospice thoughtfully addresses the whole range of each individual's physical and psychological needs in an open and honest, caring and loving way.

Most of all, hospice provides the unique opportunity that when the body can no longer be healed—we focus instead on the responsibility of bringing about healing of the spirit and healing of the soul.

23

And, in the End …

The final plan

Many of us fear that even discussing funeral plans will somehow hasten the date.

Of course, that's a myth. These family discussions certainly don't hasten the date and, most importantly, they don't give power to death and dying. The reverse is true: An honest, open discussion can lessen the fearful power of death and help you regain some control of this deeply emotional milestone. Talking and planning helps people to realistically grapple with what can be a traumatic turning point for the entire family.

Helping families to discuss these issues is a crucial role for clergy, who know that most people initially are resistant to such a discussion. Sadly, it is often only after a funeral that families realize how much stress and strife they could have prevented if they had simply talked about the funeral plans with their loved one before the time came.

Overall, the following recommendations are shared by clergy of all denominations and faiths. Two thirds of Americans say they currently have a Christian affiliation—and the portion of the U.S. population with a general Christian background is even higher than that. Each person's religious experience is unique, and each denomination varies, as well. Orthodox and Catholic practices differ from Protestant customs. Jewish, Muslim, Buddhist and Hindu communities all have their own traditional approaches to memorializing a life.

However, from a family's perspective, the issues are almost universal: How do we approach death? Let's start with three scenarios to illustrate common situations. Perhaps you may see your family in one of them.

Scenario 1: A family patriarch is diagnosed with a terminal brain tumor. Some weeks before his death, one of the daughters asks a faith leader to sit down with her siblings and her father to discuss the funeral. The faith leader welcomes this opportunity and tries to schedule a time, but the oldest son intervenes and simply says, "I don't want to upset Dad at this time." Even the idea of holding such a discussion sparks such an argument among the siblings that no meeting is held.

Then, when the father dies, the family's anxiety spills into a torrent of frantic phone calls: "What do we do about—?"

"Who does—?"

"How does—?"

"What would Dad have wanted for—?"

"Where should—?"

Scenario 2: A family matriarch is facing a major surgery that she may not survive. She calls a pastor from her hospital room and asks the pastor to bring a notebook. When the pastor arrives, she tells the pastor her life story, names her favorite hymns, describes her favorite passages from the Bible and lists several other details she would like to have included in her funeral service.

One day later, the whole family is overjoyed when the surgery is successful! Everyone is focused on rehab and a return to home. No need to discuss a funeral any further. However, the pastor keeps those notes on file. Perhaps the pastor is called to serve a different church in a different state. A good pastor will carefully preserve such files and pass them along to the newly arriving clergy. One day, those notes are sure to be both comforting and reassuring to that family.

Scenario 3: A young woman in her early 30s who has just taken part in the funeral of her father with very little advance planning winds up calling on her imam a couple of weeks later.

"I never want to experience that kind of emotional tug-of-war in our family again," she says. "We made that a lot more painful by

refusing to talk about things in advance." She hands the imam an
envelope. "I don't know what the others will do, but I decided to
write down some of my own wishes and I want you to hold onto
them until someday—I hope someday far in the future."

What all of these scenarios have in common is a call to a clergyper-
son. So, what about those families who don't know one? These days,
millions of Americans are either unaffiliated with a congregation
or have only the most tenuous connection to one. When a family
member dies, the centuries-old tradition of calling in clergy often is
skipped in favor of a more convenient call to a local funeral home.
Nationwide, these facilities are known for having good, long-standing relationships with local clergy. Often, they help families without
a home congregation to make that important clergy connection.

However, going to a funeral home without any consultation with a
faith leader can wind up focusing the entire process on the commerce
that comes after death. The list of questions begins with:

- Choosing burial or cremation
- Choosing a casket or urn
- Identifying and perhaps purchasing a plot
- Choosing a grave marker
- Drafting a paid death notice
- Ordering "sympathy cards"
- Deciding whether there will be collages of photos, a display
  of memorabilia, a video presentation—and who will produce
  this media

The list goes on and on: flowers, food, limos, death certificates, etc.

The most important lesson here for families is: Discuss these issues
early.

Going to a funeral home without any preparation is very much
like going to purchase a car without any idea of what you want or
need. The choices a family has to make can be overwhelming, especially because they may come within hours of a death.

And, that's not all. These days, a growing number of older
Americans actually take it upon themselves to visit a funeral home
and plan for future services themselves—sometimes without telling

family members. These services often are called "preneed" plans. They are common nationwide. Many families have found them to be comforting and convenient. Others have encountered problems, ranging from a plan that will not transfer later to the loved one's final location—to family disagreements about the cost and details.

One national consumer advocate advises:

- Do research on these pre-paid plans. The Federal Trade Commission regulates some aspects of these plans. Also, individual states have their own legal requirements and protections.
- Discuss this with your family. Talking openly about these issues is the most important advice throughout this chapter.
- Ask about what happens if you move, if you wish to cancel the plan entirely, or if your life circumstances change in major ways.
- Take the time to learn about the reputation of the company, exactly what you are buying and what will happen with the money you prepay.
- Make sure all details of your arrangements are shared with a person you trust.

A preneed visit to a funeral home can be part of a family's plan—but we stress it's only one possibility and one part of a family's preparation. Most people expect much more than these pragmatic details at the end of life.

So, let's return to those three scenarios, all of which involve calling clergy—the first step countless families have taken when facing death down through the centuries. Here's another important checklist:

- First—What is the religious affiliation and is there any connection with a congregation or clergy? Family members who gather around a dying relative may not share the same religious traditions. They may not appreciate how much a local congregation, or the pastoral care of clergy, means to the dying person. Even if your first call is to a funeral home, rather than clergy, the funeral home staff will ask this question immediately.

Other questions often asked by faith leaders are:

- What is the person's name?
- Favorite scripture?
- Favorite music?

Why is the person's name on this list? That should be obvious—but often isn't. What's in a name? Often, an entire world of community connections! Getting a person's name wrong can leave an indelible ache in mourners' memories. Getting it right can spark warm and loving associations.

Think about these scenarios: The current clergy in your home congregation may not know your full name. With advances in health care, people often die in their 80s or 90s and, at that point, may not have been able to regularly attend their home congregation for many years. When the family contacts that home church, a new pastor may respond who barely knows the person who has died. Most clergy are trying their best to provide compassionate care but they may be looking at a name on a membership list that was entered many years ago. For a moment, think about Joan M. Swanson. The pastor has no idea that "everyone" calls her by her middle name Marie. Then, Marie actually remarried in her 60s and now goes by Marie Peterson. In the hospital registration, she's listed as Joan Peterson. In making a hospital visit during her final days, the pastor is looking for Joan Swanson. Pastors often have trouble finding the right room because of variations in names. Then, when planning a service and providing pastoral care to the family, it helps to know that she's actually "Marie" or "Grandma Marie" to people who love her. And, of course, it helps to know that "everyone" in her assisted-living facility knows her as "Dot," because that's a nickname she picked up "years ago" in a weekly service club that makes blankets for the homeless.

So, correctly explaining your name to clergy and funeral home professionals is important—as are nicknames—because those favorite expressions link to important life stories.

Why should we ask about favorite scripture? Of course, funeral rituals vary depending on one's faith, but nearly everyone expects scripture to be read at a funeral. Clergy want to know what passages hold a powerful meaning in that person's life. Especially if the service includes a eulogy or sermon, the pastor's talk will be much more meaningful if there are favorite sections of scripture to explore.

There's another value in asking about scripture, long before there is any concern about the end of life. Having a conversation about favorite scripture is a wonderful doorway into talking with a family member about the role of faith in their life—and it will become a rich part of eventually planning for a funeral. It's an easy and often an inspiring conversation to have with a person you love. Often, family members don't think of inquiring and that leaves clergy relying on passages selected by well-meaning family members who have their own preferences. The most powerful funeral services involve a direct connection to scripture from the person we are memorializing. So, ask about scripture. It's an easy question and you are likely to enjoy the conversation.

Music? Traditions vary, but almost everyone expects music at a funeral. This is another great doorway into the life of a loved one. Just ask: "Mom, what are your favorite hymns?" You may be surprised at the wonderful insights in the conversation that unfolds. As you talk about music, remember to ask about the specific versions of a song. Most hymns have multiple verses. Some traditional songs have been updated over the centuries. The most emotive, powerful and personal moments in a funeral often revolve around music. There are many options: Someone singing a solo, the congregation singing a hymn or even the dynamic chords from an organ providing an instrumental version. All can allow pent-up emotions to come out. Such carefully chosen music evokes an enduring reminder of the person who has died.

Going over this basic list with your caregiver ensures the service will be meaningful—and it helps to avoid arguments in the midst of the emotional days that follow a death. When a friend or relative suddenly confronts your family with a song they want to sing, a different speaker than the one the family has scheduled, a reading they insist they should add—they can simply answer: "Thank you. But we talked about all of this with him—and we're doing what he wanted." End of discussion.

Then, there's one more important issue to consider before our final checklist. If the person who has died is part of a religious tradition, let clergy guide your family through the appropriate rituals. Faiths all have established traditions, which are listed in official guides for worship approved in each denomination. Many are centuries old. Clergy have the flexibility to adapt these services, which sometimes are called liturgies—but a funeral traditionally is a worship service. These are sacred moments, echoing centuries of tradition. For example, the text of the service in the United Methodist Book of Worship begins: "We have gathered here to praise God and to witness to our faith as we celebrate the life of _____. We come together in grief, acknowledging our human loss. May God grant us grace, that in pain we may find comfort, in sorrow hope, in death resurrection."

Just as weddings have been widely adapted in our current culture, families often want to adapt end-of-life services. If so, ask your clergy or funeral director about the wider range of options, including wakes and memorial services that are more generally focused on recalling and honoring a person's life. In Jewish tradition, a lot of the most important conversations and storytelling takes place during *shiva*, a week-long mourning period held in a family's home.

If you are able to respond to the basic questions already raised in this chapter, you will be well on your way toward a meaningful service. Additional conversation only adds to the confidence and comfort in the process.

Here's one last checklist of some other items you may want to discuss:

- Casket or cremation. If a casket, do you have one picked out? If cremation, do you wish to be interred, will your family wish to keep your ashes or do you wish to have your ashes scattered? There is a huge range in costs for these services. Also, remember: Religious traditions vary in their stances on these practices.

- Location of cemetery. Do you have a plot purchased or does one need to be purchased? Find out if a vault is required in your state and in the specific cemetery. Where are other family members buried—or where are they likely to wind up

in the future? Will it be easy for family members and friends
to visit on certain holidays? Also, many religious groups can
recommend locations.

- Grave marker. Again, there is a wide range of costs. There
  also may be restrictions about the size and shape of markers
  at your cemetery. What information will be included? Has
  everyone checked all the spellings and dates? Also, people
  often have a symbol they would like to see on a marker;
  sometimes, they prefer specific wording. Many grave markers
  now include illustrations as well.

- List of family members and friends. This is a vital step in
  ensuring that the next steps in your planning, especially the
  death notice, doesn't omit anyone. It's easy to forget names in
  an emotionally charged moment of crisis. People remember
  for a long time whether they were included in these final
  tributes.

- Obituary or paid death notice. It is important to distinguish
  between obituaries and paid death notices, even if you hear
  people using the terms interchangeably. In many communities
  still served by a local newspaper, newsrooms report obituaries
  of notable people—news stories reported by the staff at no
  charge to the family. Sometimes, even national newspapers
  like *The New York Times* will report obituaries on remarkable
  men and women. Obituaries are increasingly rare, however,
  because newspaper staffs are dwindling. These days, it is far
  more common for funeral home professionals to guide the
  family in writing a paid death notice. The staff often provides
  an easy-to-follow template, then makes sure the paid death
  notice appears in any local media and online. Note: These are
  just the two most common kinds of memorial texts. There are
  many other ways that biographies and eulogies can be shared.
  The family may want to print something in a sympathy card
  or funeral-service program—or place material in popular
  online websites that specialize in memorials.

- Is this a military funeral? If so, you will want to let the funeral
  home know quickly, especially if you wish to be buried at
  a national cemetery or want to have a military presence at

the memorial. Scheduling may even be beyond your control as the funeral home and the national cemetery will have to coordinate that aspect.

- Members of fraternal groups. If you are an active member of a group, they may want to send representatives to the funeral home, perhaps to perform a brief ritual. There are many groups like this. Among the most common are Masons, The American Legion, B'nai B'rith, Loyal Order of Moose, Veterans of Foreign Wars and Knights of Columbus.

- Members of sororal groups. There are many women's organizations active today, including Daughters of the American Revolution, Red Hat Society, the Junior League, Daughters of the Nile and many Greek life organizations.

- Clothing. The most common question is: What outfit should be sent to the funeral home? If the person was in the military, do they wish to be buried in uniform? A firefighter, police officer, etc. might have the same questions. Don't forget jewelry. Will they be buried with their wedding ring, watch, or favorite necklace?

- Favorite photos. This is an almost universal end-of-life ritual, now, involving many images that can be displayed at the memorial service and can be incorporated into a digital photo montage. However, you may want to have a family discussion about selecting the primary photo that will be used in any obituary, death notice or memorial folder printed for the service.

- Charities and donations. One powerful way that family and friends can honor someone is by donating to a church, charity or other organization that is close to the heart of the family. Some men and women specify such charitable giving in their will. One way to start this discussion is to ask about advance giving. Many organizations and nonprofits have helpful literature and professionals who can discuss this with families. Listing charitable contributions is a great way to help people express their grief by helping others in your honor.

Finally, don't be afraid to have this conversation. It may be a hard one; and there may be objections to talking about it. Those objections may come from the person who is elderly—or from that person's children and friends. Whichever side is showing resistance—don't give up. If you need to compassionately retreat from the subject on one occasion—bring it up the next time you are together.

When death arrives, your family will be emotional and hard-pressed to keep everything straight in their minds from conversations over the years. By putting this kind of a list together you can offer them so much help even though you aren't around.

A funeral is a sacred moment in someone's life—and this plan may be the last one you'll make. The more prepared you are to face it, the better your legacy will go forth into the lives of the men, women and children who come to mark this milestone.

About the Authors

All of our authors helped to shape this book, contributing ideas and helping us to perfect the final manuscript. All of us worked collaboratively for a year on this project. In addition, the authors agreed to serve as primary contributors on chapters within their own areas of expertise.

Emma Banze is an attorney, researcher and writer with GXG, a company that specializes in helping organizations to overcome barriers to growth. Her background also includes study of end-of-life issues and she contributed Chapter 21: Our Story, Our Legacy.

Dmitri Barvinok is Production Director of Front Edge Publishing and supervised the editing and design of this book. He is also an expert on emerging forms of media in publishing. He contributed to Chapter 7: Going Online, Chapter 12: Home Safe Home and Chapter 20: Enjoying Life.

Najah Bazzy is the founder of Zaman International, a nonprofit that offers a wide range of services for at-risk families, especially households headed by women with children. She has been honored as both a CNN network and People magazine hero. She is nationally known as an expert in transcultural nursing. She contributed Chapter 6: Saging, Not Aging.

Lisa Brown is a writer, former Congressional and Government Relations professional, life-long advocate and community lay leader dedicated to protecting and empowering women, children and the elderly. She helped enact and implement national legislation for women, children and the elderly; developed innovative child welfare, young leadership and community service initiatives; and has served on numerous philanthropic boards.

Missy Buchanan is an educator, best-selling author and nationally known advocate for the needs of aging men and women. She is a sought-after speaker for workshops and conferences and appeared twice on *Good Morning America* after helping host Robin Roberts' mother Lucimarian co-author the 2012 memoir, *My Story, My Song*. She wrote this book's Foreword.

David Crumm is founding Editor of Front Edge Publishing and *ReadTheSpirit.com* online magazine. He served as general editor of this book, working with all of the book's collaborators for a year to develop the final array of chapters.

Elisa Di Bendetto and **Larbi Megari** are journalists based in Italy and Algeria, respectively. They are co-managing directors of the International Association of Religion Journalists. They conducted the global research reflected in Chapter 10: Connecting with a Congregation, work that was sponsored by the Academy of Religion Data Archives.

Charles Ensminger is a United Methodist pastor serving the Allen Memorial United Methodist Church in Athens, Tennessee. He also is an educator, consultant and author of the earlier book, *Crafting the Sermon: A Beginner's Guide to Preaching*. He contributed Chapter 23: And in the End.

Joe Grimm is a journalism professor at Michigan State University's School of Journalism. He established a series of classes that, each year, publish guides to greater cultural competence. Grimm's students collectively have become known as the Bias Busters. Over the years, they have produced widely used books explaining racial, religious, cultural, occupational and generational groups. He was responsible for Chapter 19: Our Relationships.

Ruth Rashid Kaleniecki is a nonprofit leader and consultant, an expert in fund development and project management—and was the convener of the coalition in southeast Michigan that devoted 2020 to focusing on innovative ideas to encourage healthy aging in place. That effort included production of this book for which she served as an overall supervisor. She also serves as executive director of the Interfaith Health and Hope Coalition in the Detroit area. In addition, she contributed this book's Introduction, Chapter 1: You Are Not Alone and Meet Our Community Partners.

Joseph Krakoff is a rabbi and the Senior Director of the Jewish Hospice and Chaplaincy Network in West Bloomfield, MI. He is an educator, consultant and author of the books, *Never Long Enough: Finding Comfort and Hope Amidst Grief and Loss* and the related *Never Long Enough: Coloring/Workbook*. He contributed Chapter 22: What Is Hospice Care?

Jessica Linville is a social worker and Director of Community Based Programs at Wolverine Human Services in Michigan. She holds a Master's in Hospice and Palliative Studies with a concentration and certification in bereavement and a Master's in Social Work. She is a Licensed Social Worker. She also has worked with children, families and older adults for many years. She helped to coordinate this book project and contributed Chapter 15: Dress for Success, and Chapter 17: A Trip to the Doctor.

Patricia Montemurri is a nationally award-winning journalist who reported for many years for *The Detroit Free Press*. She also has written a series of books about Michigan's religious communities, including *Blessed Solanus Casey* and *Immaculate Heart of Mary Sisters of Michigan*. She contributed Chapter 13: Emergency Preparedness.

Benjamin Pratt is a retired United Methodist pastor and counselor whose expertise over many years led him to write the *Guide for Caregivers* among other inspirational books about overcoming the many challenges of contemporary life. He contributed Chapter 8: Caring for Our Caregivers.

Mary Rumman is a social worker who works within the University of Michigan Healthcare System and specializes in helping older men and women and their families cope with the many challenges of aging. She contributed Chapter 18: Directing Our Care.

Meet Our Community Partners

This book came to be, as so many things do, through a meeting of the minds of organizations—nonprofits in and around metropolitan Detroit, Michigan. Leaders from these organizations came together believing that things could be better for the elders among us and for those who care for them.

In summer 2019, several organizations committed to working together to improve the state of healthy aging in Detroit. Without knowing specifically what that meant or what it would look like, the nonprofits agreed to work together through a grant to develop a plan to improve the quality of life for seniors in Detroit.

Understanding that much of what is experienced in Detroit isn't unique to our region, the organizations also decided to work on a guide to healthy aging. We wanted a resource that people could use to better understand the things about aging in America that most of us don't know—until we suddenly *need* to know them. This healthy aging guide would be grounded in Detroit, but inform a national audience.

In late 2019, funding was approved, and the resulting Agencies United for Healthy Aging was born. This coalition met monthly, developed working groups, conducted interviews, and began identifying the barriers to healthy aging in Detroit.

Unexpectedly, in the March 2020 rise of COVID-19, the meetings became video conferences and the workgroups focused on food distribution mechanisms. The leaders from the organizations supported each other through the months of the pandemic as Detroit was one of the hardest hit cities in the world.

Through it all, the following organizations and individuals contributed to the work of Agencies United for Healthy Aging, the coalition without which this book would not have been possible:

Bridging Communities, Inc. is a grassroots organization dedicated to enhancing the quality of life for elders in the Southwest Detroit area by providing valuable resources and needed support. Serving one of the most diverse communities in Michigan, Bridging Communities is responsive to community needs, no matter if those needs are named in English, Spanish, or Arabic. Executive Director Phyllis Edwards is a master social worker in every sense who proudly and honestly starts each meeting by declaring, "It's a great day in the neighborhood!"

Brilliant Detroit is dedicated to building kid success families and neighborhoods where families with children ages 0–8 have what they need to be school ready, healthy and stable. Brilliant Detroit does this by providing proven programming and support year-round out of Brilliant Detroit homes in high-need neighborhoods. As the fiscal sponsor for the grant that funded the collaborative, Brilliant Detroit's partnership made all of this possible. Co-Founder and CEO Cindy Eggleton's community-building and transformational leadership earned her an AARP 2021 Purpose Prize Winner Award. Health Program Manager Megan Reeves came to the coalition as someone whose day job focuses on implementing health programming for children and their parents and very quickly became an advocate for seniors through her participation.

Camp Fire Southeast Michigan believes that young people want to shape the world and provides the opportunity for them to find their spark, lift their voice and discover who they are. Camp Fire joined the table to help Agencies United for Healthy Aging create opportunities for intergenerational programming and interaction, including spending time at Camp Wathana in Holly, Michigan. CEO Elizabeth Longley continually brought to the table not only her experience at Camp Fire, but her decades of experience within nonprofits and municipal government, elevating best practices from a variety of times and places.

Cody Rouge Community Action Alliance seeks to revitalize and sustain a healthy community where residents have access to and promote a high quality of life. Serving the Cody Rouge area of northwest Detroit, Cody Rouge Community Action Alliance fulfills its mission with strong support from philanthropic/corporate funders like Skillman Foundation, Kresge Foundation, Ford Foundation, General Motors, Quicken Loans and DTE. Executive Director Kenyetta Campbell and Office Manager/Executive Assistant Chanelle Ward both have deep community roots and are thriving entrepreneurs, making them powerful role models.

Detroit Area Agency on Aging is the aging and disability resource center that covers the cities of Detroit, Hamtramck, Highland Park, Harper Woods and the five Grosse Pointes. Its mission is to educate, advocate and promote healthy aging to enable people to make choices about home and community-based services and long term care that will improve their quality of life. President and CEO Ronald Taylor was a key supporter of Agencies United for Healthy Aging, recognizing that if Detroit Area Agency on Aging is going to improve the lives of elders, it needs to have deep community connections. Director of Information and Assistance Crystal Hood served as a conduit between the Area Agency on Aging and the collaborating partners, helping to ensure that communities were aware of available resources, especially during the COVID-19 pandemic.

Franian Consulting, LLC works to strengthen small- to mid-sized nonprofits by providing consulting services in fund development, strategic planning, program development and management, impact tracking, and more. Through a team of nonprofit professionals, Franian Consulting serves as an extension of its clients, filling in gaps and moving the organization forward. Owner and principal Ruth Rashid Kaleniecki is the architect of and grant director for Agencies United for Healthy Aging.

Front Edge Publishing is this book's publishing house, and also so much more. A local publisher with a conscience, Front Edge specializes in fast and flexible publishing while also engaging in content creation. Long-time journalist and co-founder David Crumm oriented us to mission-aligned projects and initiatives on the national and international landscape. Director of Production Dmitri Barvinok kept us to our timeline and assured us that we would end up with a product of which we would all be proud. (He was right!)

GenesisHOPE CDC is a community development organization that strives to improve the quality of life for those living and working in the Islandview/Greater Villages on Detroit's east side. It is a place where opportunity is vast and hope is plentiful. GenesisHOPE engages residents, local businesses, institutions and other change makers in the equitable development of healthy resilient communities by promoting healthy living, empowering financial health, and providing affordable living and open green spaces. Executive Director Jeanine Hatcher has served as a champion for addressing the social determinants of health through systems and policy change, driving the agenda for the inclusion of community health workers as a key piece of what should be our response to racial health disparities. Community Relationship Coordinator Jennine Spencer has been a mouthpiece for individual seniors in desperate need of assistance.

Interfaith Health and Hope Coalition seeks to unite and empower communities of faith and health organizations in order to improve individual and community health through partnership-building, education and advocacy, with a special emphasis on the uninsured and underserved. The Coalition cultivates a network of interconnected faith-based, health care organizations that work together to build capacity for strong healthy communities, providing health education and social policy information, advocacy, increasing access to health services, and promoting wellness. Executive Director Ruth Rashid Kaleniecki, with support from Onoriode Emmanuel Ekokotu, Lauren Howling and Amanda Nihem, worked to ensure that faith communities were represented at the table and that the important role that they play in the lives of countless elders was recognized.

Michigan Health Endowment Fund awarded the grant that has funded this work. The Health Fund's mission is to improve the health of Michigan residents, with special emphasis on the health and wellness of children and seniors, while reducing the cost of health care. Director of Healthy Aging Kari Sederburg has been a critical thought partner in the project, connecting the stakeholders with other relevant efforts and initiatives in Metro Detroit and beyond.

Mission Lift was hired as the external evaluator for Agencies United for Healthy Aging, but became much more of a partner in the process. As a Detroit-based agency that has worked with more than 100 nonprofit clients throughout its history, Mission Lift has deep grounding in the work. Mission Lift's founder Janet Ray reminded us of what she and her team heard from seniors they interviewed, keeping us focused on the needs that they articulated. Staffer Maria Schmeider skillfully managed record-keeping, reporting and data presentation to tell the story of the group's work.

Sinai-Grace Guild Community Development Corporation evolved from the Grace Guild of Sinai-Grace Hospital, serving patients and residents in Northwest Detroit. Since its 2015 community visioning process that led to its renaming, Sinai-Grace Guild has been driven by community residents, businesses and leaders and is committed to holistic and equitable revitalization toward a thriving, healthy and sustainable Northwest Detroit. Executive Director Lisa Campbell and Program Manager Crystal Head have dug into the work, sharing their experiences to help make all of Detroit a healthier place for seniors to live.

Urban Aging News is a free quarterly publication focused on metro Detroit. A wonderful resource for seniors and caregivers alike, the paper includes both timely journalism and information about available community resources. Through its engagement in Agencies United for Healthy Aging, Urban Aging News was connected with seniors in the communities served by the other partners and featured their varied stories, lifting up the wide range of experiences of aging for the readership. Publisher Patricia Ann Rencher has greatly contributed to the work of Agencies United for Healthy Aging, offering full access to her decades of experience as a senior advocate.

Agencies United for Healthy Aging has also benefitted from time with guest presenters, including Dan Wojciak, Staff Attorney and MI Health Link Ombudsman with the Michigan Elder Justice Initiative and Sarah Slocum, Co-Director of the Program to Improve Eldercare within the Center for Appropriate Care at Altarum.

Acknowledgments

This book would not have been possible without the commitment of the partners listed in the Meet Our Community Partners section. Their grounding in the communities that they serve provided context and a rich landscape of experiences from which to grow the strategy to improve healthy aging. Their passion and candor was equaled only by their resilience and perseverance as they worked tirelessly to meet the evolving needs of their community throughout the COVID-19 pandemic.

The book's contributing authors are listed with their short biographies in About the Authors. The words, reflections and experience of this broad range of experts make this book what it is—a helpful resource for those who need to know more about how to navigate life's later years.

Early readers who helped to shape the final book included Jessica Linville, Ruth Rashid Kaleniecki, Patricia Rencher, Jerry Sloan, Dan Wojciak and many others, including all of the contributing authors. Their feedback and comments helped create what you see before you. Of course, we also want to thank the Front Edge Publishing team: David Crumm, Dmitri Barvinok, Susan Stitt, Patty Thompson, John Hile, Celeste Dykas, and Rick Nease.

Now What?

For more information about this book and the authors, visit the resource page at www.HealthyAgingBook.com. You will also find news and updates about our ongoing work with readers—including the release in 2021 of a discussion guide for the book.

Contact us directly at info@FrontEdgePublishing.com to learn more about:

- How to place bulk orders for the book.
- How to order specially modified editions of the book that can include your organization's logo.
- How to provide feedback for future editions of the book.
- Ideas for using this book in community outreach programs in your region.

Proceeds from this book support ongoing work with our partnering nonprofits on encouraging healthy aging in place. See the Meet Our Community Partners page for more information.

CPSIA information can be obtained
at www.ICGtesting.com
Printed in the USA
BVHW032123060421
604336BV00009B/1070

9 781641 800952